"This is a MUST READ for all mental and health care providers that take care of women with pelvic or sexual pain – any provider that truly wants to make a difference in their patient or client's life."

**Lynn Wang, MD, FACOG, CSC, CSE**;
*Main Line Health, PA, USA*

"An essential read for any provider who works with people experiencing intimate pain or with a history of trauma. The combination of research, medical explanations and poignant patient stories creates a great primer for a very complex and important topic."

**Dana Shanis, MD, FACOG,**
*Ob/Gyn and Owner of VHealth & Wellness, Philadelphia, PA, USA*

"Davidson confronts the normalization of women's sexual pain, pelvic pain and trauma and its profound impact on a woman's quality of life. She unpacks the layers of a woman's pelvic pain journey that too often go unseen or are dismissed. Boldly naming the many ways women are underserved and failed by their institutional systems, this book provides a strong call-to-action for institutions and professionals, along with a comprehensive and proven interdisciplinary treatment approach, to help women heal from trauma, pain and cultural betrayal."

**Carolynn Aristone, MSW, LCSW, CST,**
*Founder and Executive Director of the Center for Intimate Relationships, L.L.C, USA*

# EFFECTIVE TREATMENT OF WOMEN'S PELVIC AND SEXUAL PAIN DISORDERS

This book presents a comprehensive overview of pelvic and sexual pain disorders in women and equips therapists to treat these issues in a culturally sensitive way, examining the link between unwanted sexual experiences and the development of sexual pain in later life.

Drawing on the wealth of recent research acknowledging the increased risk of developing a pelvic/sexual pain disorder in women who have experienced sexual trauma, Heather Lauren Davidson offers a much-needed resource for professionals within the essential context of the #MeToo movement. Chapters address a range of topics, including types of sexual pain disorders, disparities in the mental health system that affect women's access to treatment, how to establish treatment goals for individuals and couples, and effective relapse prevention plans. Illustrated throughout by vignettes and case studies, the book addresses a lack of knowledge in assessing and treating the experiences of these women and explores in depth how they face complex difficulties in accessing diagnosis and treatment.

Guided by culturally competent assessment and the use of evidence-based treatment techniques, clinicians will learn to effectively navigate the treatment of women presenting with pelvic/sexual pain disorders and sexual trauma.

**Heather Lauren Davidson,** MA, LPC, CST, is a Licensed Professional Counselor, Certified EMDR Therapist, and Certified Sex Therapist. Heather is the owner and founder of Better Being Main Line, a counseling practice outside of Philadelphia, USA, which specializes in women's emotional and sexual wellness.

# EFFECTIVE TREATMENT OF WOMEN'S PELVIC AND SEXUAL PAIN DISORDERS

---

## Healing the Body and Mind During the #MeToo Era

*Heather Lauren Davidson*

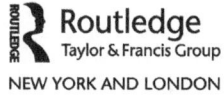

Routledge
Taylor & Francis Group

NEW YORK AND LONDON

Cover image: © Getty Images

First published 2023
by Routledge
605 Third Avenue, New York, NY 10158

and by Routledge
4 Park Square, Milton Park, Abingdon, Oxon, OX14 4RN

*Routledge is an imprint of the Taylor & Francis Group, an informa business*

© 2023 Heather Lauren Davidson

The right of Heather Lauren Davidson to be identified as author of this work has been asserted in accordance with sections 77 and 78 of the Copyright, Designs and Patents Act 1988.

*Library of Congress Cataloging-in-Publication Data*
A catalog record for this book has been requested

ISBN: 978-0-367-76716-7 (hbk)
ISBN: 978-0-367-76715-0 (pbk)
ISBN: 978-1-003-16823-2 (ebk)

DOI: 10.4324/9781003168232

Typeset in Joanna
by Apex CoVantage, LLC

For survivors
#MeToo

# CONTENTS

# ACKNOWLEDGEMENTS

I would like to sincerely thank the clients who have shared their stories with me over the years. It has been an honor to be a small part of their journeys. Their courage and resiliency are reminders for me on the days when I am feeling the most discouraged, why I continue to do this work.

I would also like to thank Ellie Duncan and Heather Evans and all others affiliated with Routledge/Taylor and Francis who have made the publication of this book possible. Also deserving of thanks are Luci Morreale for her amazing illustrations, Melissa DiGiovannantonio for her help with editing, Pete Ondish for his assistance with creating and analyzing the survey, and Stephanie Muntzer for her feedback on the medical components of the illustrations.

And finally, I would like to thank my colleagues, mentors, and supervisors who have provided guidance and training throughout the course of my career.

– HLD

# 1

# #METOO AND PELVIC/SEXUAL PAIN

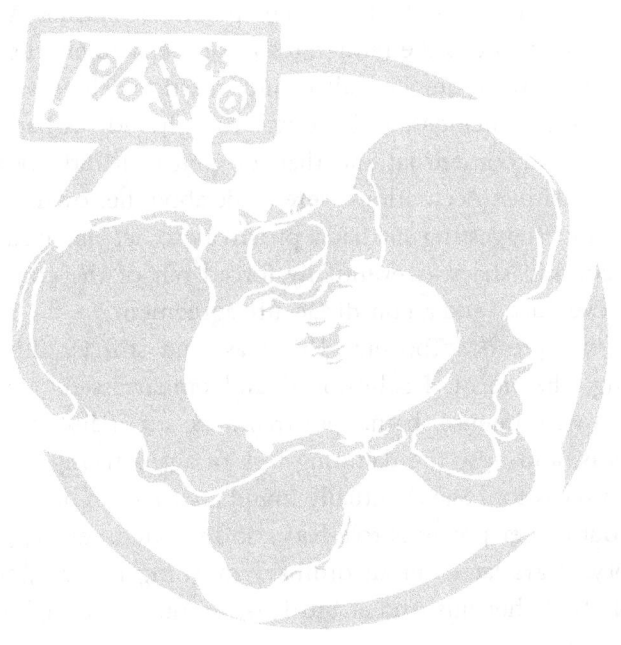

DOI: 10.4324/9781003168232-1

## Noemi and the Mental "Ping-Pong Match"

"It's like my mind keeps synching up these traumas, because they're the same. Different situations obviously, but it's the same feelings," Noemi lamented in my office. Rewind to 2009, to a young college graduate desperately searching for a job in the recession. One of the "lucky ones," she landed a solid job at an established company. Her father, a first-generation immigrant from a Latin American country, boasted to everyone he knew about her job. Noemi smiled, remembering that part fondly. She excelled at her job, and a senior member of the company took interest in her and developed a mentorship role with her. Noemi appreciated Mr. X's mentorship and believed it to be crucial in her being able to advance at the company. However, she recalled always feeling that something was "off" but ignored her bad gut feelings. About a year into the job, Mr. X coerced her into a private room at a company event and sexually assaulted her. "I tucked it away," Noemi said in reference to the assault.

After the sexual assault, she was tormented by the decision to report the incident or not. She feared for her career but also felt compelled to protect others. The rumination ate her alive. Literally. She lost nearly 15 pounds in the months following the sexual assault. After she disclosed the incident to the human resources department, her motivation and character were quickly called into question. There was an "investigation" of the incident, and she was told that Mr. X had claimed the encounter was consensual and that, of course, it did not happen at a work event either. Accusations were made about her own sexual history, with rumors suggesting she had a proclivity to lie. Her accusations were dismissed, and she was eventually forced out of the company with a small "severance" and a non-disclosure agreement.

This was pre-#MeToo era. This was, and still is, although slowly changing, the norm. Disillusioned and embarrassed, Noemi silently struggled with intense shame, posttraumatic stress disorder (PTSD)–like symptoms, and now the daunting task of again trying to secure a job during a recession. She eventually found another job but believed being forced out of her previous role had also impacted her long-term career trajectory. Years later, on an ordinary morning in 2018, sitting across the table from her husband at breakfast, scrolling through the news on her phone, she stumbled across an article confirming what she knew all along – she was not the only victim. According to the article, there were dozens. "I threw my phone across the room," she recalled.

The sexual assault was not something she had told her husband about. They had met two years after the sexual assault through mutual friends. "I remember thinking, 'What if he doesn't believe me?' Obviously, I did not have a positive experience with disclosing this before, and I didn't really find it relevant to my life at the time," she explained. So again, she tucked it away. Shortly after reading the article that made her aware of other victims at her past job, Noemi found out she was pregnant. It was something the couple had hoped for, but they had struggled to conceive. Noemi was thrilled that she was going to become a mother.

Noemi found herself "on edge" during the pregnancy. She wondered if it was related to having the memory of her sexual assault resurface or simply anxiety related to being pregnant. The birth itself went fine, but Noemi's gut told her something was off. "Before being released, I again told the doctor I didn't feel right, but everyone – my mom, my doctors, and my husband – reassured me I was okay. That it was just 'new mom jitters.' And maybe part of it was, but obviously, something went wrong at some point," she recounted. Two days after being discharged, while at home with her newborn daughter and six-year-old stepson, Noemi experienced a postpartum hemorrhage. Carefully, she placed her newborn on the floor, told her stepson to wait in his room, dialed 911 . . . "and the next thing I remember was waking up at the hospital." Elated to be alive despite needing a hysterectomy, Noemi returned home and again "tucked it away."

Months later when Noemi and her husband attempted having sex again for the first time since having the baby, she experienced sharp pain upon insertion. The experience made her feel nervous. The second time it occurred, her anxiety felt more like full-blown panic. Afterwards she started thinking about Mr. X's tight grip on her arms . . . then the blood from her hemorrhage on their wood floors . . . then the pain from when Mr. X attempted to insert a finger . . . then feeling the warm blood rushing down her legs just before she dialed 911. "It was like my mind was in a ping-pong match, back and forth and back and forth between each of those traumas. I couldn't stop thinking about either event." She began to avoid sex with her husband due to the pain with penetration, and because the pain triggered anxiety and memories, she could no longer "tuck it away."

She consulted with her OB/GYN regarding the pain with sex. The doctor told her with a big sigh and eye roll, "Well, that's just sex after having a baby. Just try to have a glass of wine and relax." Noemi burst into tears as soon as she got to her car because as she saw it, "If sex was now just going to feel like this, I wouldn't be able to have it. I couldn't take the pain, and I couldn't take those memories popping up when I needed to be focused on my kids, and my job, and my husband, who was already frustrated with me. I didn't know what I was going to do." Unfortunately, many women like Noemi who experience pain with sex are dismissed by their doctors or are told the pain is "normal."

For women who have a pelvic/sexual pain disorder and a history of sexual trauma, they often describe the two experiences as being very parallel. In both situations, they usually know that something is wrong but are told by people in positions of authority or power that they are fine or that they have misunderstood the situation. They are dismissed and sometimes even blamed. The stress of both situations feed off each other and compound both the emotional and physical pain. And despite how common pelvic/sexual pain disorders are for women and how common unwanted sexual experiences are for women, healthcare and mental health providers are profoundly ill-equipped to diagnosis and treat women with these disorders. If you work with women, you need to be able to effectively treat both presenting problems and often concurrently.

## #MeToo

Unwanted sexual experiences and their consequences have gained more attention thanks to the #MeToo movement. In 2006, Tarana Burke started "Me Too" to raise awareness about sexual assault, especially among women of color. Previously, Ms. Burke had started a nonprofit in 1997 that helped women and girls who had experienced sexual harassment and sexual assault ("Get to Know Us," 2020). The hashtag "#MeToo" went viral in October 2017 after actress Alyssa Milano encouraged via Twitter for survivors of sexual violence to tweet "#MeToo" as a way to draw attention to the magnitude of this issue (Pflum, 2018). Since then, many high-profile cases involving sexual harassment and sexual assault have been highlighted in the media.

Globally, the #MeToo movement has been embraced as evidenced by "#YoTambien" in Spain and in many other Latin American countries, "#BalanceTonPorc" in France, and "#quellavoltache" in Italy (Stone & Vogelstein, 2019; Di Caro, 2017). Since the fall of 2017, the hashtag #MeToo is used an average of 55,319 times a day on Twitter across 85 countries, with 29% of the tweets being in a language other than English (Anderson & Toor, 2020). Like the United States which continues to grapple with gender-based violence, many countries are facing their own reckoning regarding sexual violence against women. Over the past few years, Mexico has been experiencing rallies organized by the *revolucion diamantina* (glitter revolution), which aimed to raise awareness about violence against women, including femicides and sexual violence (Phillips, 2019). In France the *#NousToutes* (All of Us) movement is speaking out against domestic violence and gender-based violence (Rushworth, 2018; #NousToutes, 2020). Similar protests denouncing gender-based violence and sexual violence have occurred in many parts of the world in the past year, including Spain, Russia, South Arica, Sudan, Turkey, Bulgaria, Columbia, Chile, Argentina, El Salvador, and many more (Del Pozo, 2019; Oppenheim, 2019).

As a former elite athlete, of all the horrific cases in the United States highlighted in the media since the #MeToo movement, the Larry Nassar case has always particularly bothered me. The level of dedication and sacrifice young athletes need to make for the small chance that they can peak in a narrow window of time to "make it" is unfathomable to those who have not lived it. Female athletes have additional barriers, including significantly less financial support and the public's general lack of interest in women's sports. In fact, women now make up 40% of those participating in sports but only receive 4% of all sports media coverage. Of this tiny amount of coverage, the focus tends to be on women's physical appearances or personal lives rather than their athletic abilities (UNESCO, 2019). Additional barriers for women should not have to include enduring chronic sexual assault under the guise of needed medical care. Dr. Larry Nassar claimed he was using osteopathic manipulation to treat the pelvic floor, when in reality he was sexually abusing young female athletes.

Larry Nassar was a sports medicine doctor for Michigan State University and USA Gymnastics. Extremely well known in his field and touted as an expert in osteopathic manipulation, Nassar had access to hundreds of young gymnasts. To date there are over 500 known victims, with the abuse having occurred over a span of three decades. Sadly, dozens of authority figures knew of the abuse for most of this time and did nothing. Despite dozens of women reporting Dr. Nassar to their coaches, athletic trainers, and even the police over decades, their reports were ignored. As Tim Evans (2018) from the *Indianapolis Star* explained, "I saw the smooth Nassar, a master manipulator who had convinced police and university officials that earlier complaints were misunderstandings, and went on molesting young girls . . . he tried to convince me the 'misunderstanding' was the result of the women's ignorance of his sophisticated medical work."

This statement highlights the damage done by the cultural belief that women do not understand or know their own bodies, hence their "confusion" about Dr. Nassar's treatment. This perception is part of what allowed Dr. Nassar to convince others in positions of power that he was innocent, and women's unawareness and naivete of their own bodies was the issue. However, even once it became clearer that Dr. Nassar was indeed sexually abusing child and teen athletes, those with this knowledge did nothing. At least four major institutions knew about the abuse and chose to do nothing, including Michigan State University, USA Gymnastics, the US Olympic Committee, and Twistars Gymnastics. According to *Detroit News*, at least 14 officials at Michigan State were aware of Nassar's abuse two decades before his arrest. Some victims were threatened by USA Gymnastics to remain quiet. The FBI "investigated" the reported abuses yet did nothing (Hauser & Astor, 2018; Cohen & Shenk, 2020). While Larry Nassar was certainly a monster, so were the adults who enabled his behavior.

Rachel Denhollander, the first victim to file a criminal complaint, stated:

> A monster was stopped last year, after decades of being allowed to prey on women and little girls, and he wasn't stopped by a single person who could have, and should have, stopped him at least 20 years

ago. He was stopped by the victims, who had to fight through being silenced, being threatened, being mocked, by the officials at MSU (Michigan State University) who they appealed to for help. And now the very people who should have been protecting us all along . . . have thumbed their nose at any semblance of accountability.

(Kozlowski, 2018)

There have always been monsters. There will always be monsters. But how different would things be for girls and women if we actually listened to them when they say, "Someone is hurting me"? Or similarly, if we listened to them when they say, "My body is hurting"?

## Sexual Assault and Pelvic/Sexual Pain: Parallel Experiences

And just as survivors of sexual abuse are dismissed and are told they misunderstood what has happened, women with pelvic pain disorders often experience something very similar when seeking diagnosis and treatment. Commonly, my clients tell me that healthcare providers dismiss their concerns or tell them that their symptoms do not warrant investigation or treatment. Some research studies have demonstrated the impact of such interactions. In the case of endometriosis, for instance, women see on average eight different doctors over 10 years before receiving a diagnosis (McCoy Cohn, 2016). Sadly, in this time, many women are living with extreme chronic pain, and the disease progresses further, jeopardizing their future fertility and negatively impacting their ability to complete school, participate in the workforce, engage in enjoyable hobbies, and achieve financial stability. What if the first doctor, or even the third doctor, listened and responded when a female patient told them about their severe period pain or pain with sex? It is possible that they would be able to get a diagnosis years sooner, making the disease much more manageable because it would not have as much time to progress. Their quality of life would be better, and the disease would not have so broadly impacted other areas of their life.

Culturally, we have a problem. We do not listen to girls or women when they say, "Someone is hurting me," or "My body is hurting."

Instead, we tell them they do not understand their own bodies, that they are not the authorities on their own bodies. We tell them they have a low pain tolerance, or they misunderstood their perpetrator's intentions. We tell them that perhaps they are to blame for the abuse or pelvic/sexual pain. Sadly, I believe as a society, we prime women for these messages from a very young age. Just as the young female gymnasts became habituated to abuse, I think many girls in our culture experience something similar, albeit on a smaller scale. Jennifer Sey, former US National Team member for women's gymnastics, stated in Netflix's documentary *Athlete A* (2020):

> You know, in other sports, the athletes are adults. They can reasonably make choices about what they want. I don't think that is true in gymnastics. These kids go to these national training centers when they're ten years old. They are abused and mistreated, for years, so even by the time they're of age, the line between tough coaching and child abuse, gets blurred. So, then when real obvious abuse, sexual abuse, happens, you already don't believe your own take on things. Because you think you're hungry, you think your ankle hurts, you think that you're working really hard, and you're screamed at that you're lazy and you're fat and there's nothing wrong with your ankle. I can only imagine that what you feel is, I'm lucky to be here, so I'm not going to say anything.

Unwanted sexual experiences are very common for women in the United States, and many women experience multiple occurrences of sexual violence. Let's consider risk over the course of a woman's life in the United States. Before age 18, there is a one in four chance she will be sexually abused (Stoltenborgh et al., 2015). If she attends college, she has a 26.4% chance of being raped or sexually assaulted (Cantor et al., 2020). Once in the workplace, she may be part of the 25% to 85% of women having experienced sexual harassment while working (Golshan, 2017). Even if she is not sexually harassed at work, chances are she will experience street harassment. Street harassment continues to be prevalent in the United States with 65% of women reporting street harassment in which 23% had also been touched sexually, 20% had been followed, and 9% forced do engage in an unwanted sexual experience (Kearl, 2014).

And overall, one in every five women in the United States has been a victim of rape, with 10% having been raped by a partner and 8% of rapes occurring in the workplace (Black et al., 2011; Duhart, 2001). Not great odds for women in the United States.

Unwanted sexual experiences are traumatic, but the context in which they occur and the responses by those around them can compound this trauma. Jennifer J. Freyd from the University of Oregon coined the term "institutional betrayal." Institutional betrayal is "wrongdoings perpetrated by an institution upon individuals dependent on that institution, including failure to prevent or respond supportively to wrongdoings by individuals (e.g. sexual assault) committed within the context of the institution" (Freyd, 2021). So, for instance, in the Larry Nassar case, not only did the young gymnasts endure sexual trauma, but they also experienced institutional betrayal. The institutions responsible for the safety of the young gymnasts completely failed them. Even when authorities at the highest levels of these institutions learned of the abuse, they chose to protect the abuser and enabled him in continuing to abuse young women.

Institutional betrayal is extremely important for clinicians to be familiar with, as it creates another level of trauma, can prolong the trauma in cases of ongoing abuse and increase the chances of negative outcomes such as developing PTSD or experiencing suicidality. Women who have experienced sexual trauma commonly experience institutional betrayal. For instance, 46% of college students who were sexually victimized in an institutional context also report experiences of institutional betrayal (Smith & Freyd, 2013). Institutional betrayal is one layer of betrayal that survivors experience, but I believe there are many levels of betrayal that exacerbate survivors' trauma symptoms and complicate their recoveries. Survivors may experience additional betrayals in the form of dismissing the survivor's experience; failing to provide emotional, psychological, or financial support; or engaging in victim blaming by partners, family, friends, or colleagues.

Having a pelvic/sexual pain disorder can be a very distressing experience and is sometimes traumatic. And often, what I hear from my pelvic/sexual pain clients over and over is that responses from others or lack of response from others, especially doctors or people in positions of authority whom the client perceives could help, exacerbates the distress. Being directly told or implied that they do not know or understand their bodies and then continuing to suffer the long-term consequences of a pelvic/ sexual pain disorder because of the failure to provide needed medical treatment and care mirrors the institutional betrayal that survivors of sexual violence experience. In addition, my clients with pelvic/sexual pain often experience similar interpersonal betrayals as the survivors of sexual violence.

"It is bad enough having pelvic pain, but honestly, what has been equally as worse for me has been the years of no one believing me," explained Violet, a 28-year-old biracial woman who had entered therapy for anxiety. Most of what was driving Violet's anxiety, however, was from living with debilitating chronic pelvic pain. Shortly after Violet got her period at age 13, she started to experience severe pelvic pain with her period along with other disruptive symptoms that interfered with her ability to focus in school. Despite Violet and her mother's both express- ing concern about these symptoms to Violet's doctors over the years, they were dismissed. Violet's mom began to dismiss her, too: "The doctors said you're okay. You need to toughen up. It's just a period." Like many women with endometriosis, Violet was written off as a young woman with a low pain tolerance who was simply making a big deal out of her period. This is an example of institutional betrayal – the healthcare sys- tem's total failure to respond to a young woman repeatedly seeking help for painful and disruptive symptoms. Violet did not have some complex mystery illness; rather, she had one of the most common reproductive diseases that impacts an estimated 10% of all women.

As a transplant to the northeast for graduate school, Violet finally saw an endometriosis specialist who performed a laparoscopic surgery and confirmed the suspected diagnosis. Sadly, by the time Violet received this diagnosis, 13 years had passed, and her endometriosis had spread to many different organs and systems in her body. The doctor even removed one of her ovaries during the surgery because it was riddled with endo- metriosis adhesions, and she was told given the amount of scarring in her uterus from the endometriosis adhesions, it would be highly unlikely that she would be able to have children of her own. Like many trauma survivors, when it came to diagnosing and getting treatment for her pel- vic pain condition, the system had failed her. I also believe a type of institutional betrayal occurs for women seeking diagnosis and treatment for pelvic/sexual pain conditions. These dismissals of women's complaints and delays in treatment have significant consequences to their lives and sadly parallel their experiences with unwanted sexual experiences, which many of them have.

We know that unwanted sexual experiences have been associated with a number of physical health issues, including depression, anxiety, eating disorders, PTSD, addiction, injury, chronic pain, disability, cardiovascular disease, and disruptive menopause symptoms (Gibson et al., 2018; Miller et al., 2018). Interestingly enough, some studies are also connecting unwanted sexual experiences with a greater risk of developing a pelvic/sexual pain disorder. Multiple studies have demonstrated that adolescent girls and adult women with genito-pelvic pain disorders are more likely to report sexual abuse and severe physical abuse than women without genito-pelvic pain (Harlow & Stewart, 2005; Khandker et al., 2014; Landry & Bergeron, 2011). Compared with women with genito-pelvic pain who did not report sexual abuse, women with genito-pelvic pain and a history of sexual abuse were also found to have significantly lower levels of sexual functioning and psychological adjustment (Leclerc et al., 2010). Another study found that many forms of childhood maltreatment were associated with lower sexual functioning and higher anxiety. It also found that women and their partners' reports of childhood maltreatment were associated with higher affective pain for women with vulvodynia (Corsini-Munt et al., 2016).

These studies remind me of a question I try to keep in mind during the assessment of women presenting for pelvic/sexual pain: "What is the pelvis holding?" (Figure 1.1). For Violet, it was the feeling of "never being good enough." As a biracial woman growing up in rural Tennessee, she often felt like she did not fit in. In college, it was the same feeling, but then it was also highlighted by coming from a much less privileged place than many of her peers. During college, she was sexually assaulted by someone she viewed as a friend, and she felt as though no one would believe her. When she did finally muster up the courage to disclose to her college about the sexual assault, she was dismissed and lectured about binge drinking. As the years passed and the doctors shuffled her along from one to the next, she could not help but wonder, "What is it about me that no one ever believes me? Is it because they can't figure out 'what I am' because I'm poor? A woman? Why am I not good enough to be believed?"

I once pitched the question of "What is your pelvis holding?" to Paula, and she quickly shot back, "A big ball of shame." Paula, a 20-year-old college student-athlete, had entered therapy as she began to question how her first romantic relationship unfolded. What initially felt like

# What is your pelvis holding?

**Financial instability**

**Childcare concerns**

**Relationship distress**

**Anxiety**

**Depression**

**Worry for family**

**Trauma**

**Burnout**

Can you think of any others?

"first love" as a teenager began to feel more sinister once she went to college. With the time and space away from her "first love," she saw the pattern of grooming and abuse. She was also experiencing pain with penetrative sex, which confused her because she "loved and trusted" her college boyfriend. For Siobhan, a 33-year-old married woman presenting to therapy with lifelong vaginismus, her pelvis was holding on to "protection." Another client, Rebecca, was unsure what her pelvis was holding but remarked that her chronic pelvic pain disorder made her body "a prison."

This book will follow five case vignettes throughout its entirety: Noemi, Paula, Rebecca, Siobhan, and Violet. These are case composites that represent the hundreds of women I have treated in therapy with pelvic/sexual pain disorders, many who also have unwanted sexual experiences in their histories. Anyone who works with women, whether in an individual or couple's counseling setting or as a healthcare provider, needs to be aware of pelvic/sexual pain disorders, unwanted sexual experiences, and the interplay between these two experiences. Both of these experiences are so common for women that I do not believe you can treat women without having basic knowledge about pelvic/sexual pain disorders and unwanted sexual experiences. This book is an in-depth guide to treating pelvic/sexual pain and unwanted sexual experiences that I hope will help to bridge the gap in care that exists in the mental health and healthcare fields.

The next chapter explores common causes of pelvic/sexual pain, including vulvodynia, pelvic floor dysfunction, endometriosis, interstitial cystitis, physical trauma, hormonal changes, uterine fibroids, vulvar skin disorders, and lack of education. Basic facts and functioning of the pelvic floor and the fascia are also highlighted. This chapter also discusses the changes in the DSM-V, which merged the previous diagnoses of vaginismus and dyspareunia into a singular diagnosis: genito-pelvic pain/penetration disorder (GPPPD). Research connecting the impact of trauma and chronic stress on pelvic/sexual pain disorders and the research on the impact of pelvic/sexual pain disorders on women's quality of life are also reviewed.

Chapter 3 serves as an overview on the research regarding on unwanted sexual experiences against women in the United States. Institutional betrayal and other forms of betrayal trauma are explored.

The chapter also discussed important considerations in working with survivors, as well as how clinicians can prevent burnout when working with trauma cases. Chapter 4 highlights how women's experiences with sexual trauma often parallel their process of trying to obtain a diagnosis or seek treatment for a pelvic/sexual pain disorder. It is because of these parallels that the two experiences can trigger and exacerbate each other. The "layers of betrayal" are identified, and examples of betrayal trauma in the medical system for women suffer from pelvic/sexual pain disorders are explored. Common barriers that women with pelvic/sexual pain disorders often face when attempting to receiving adequate healthcare are reviewed.

Chapter 5 serves as an overview of completing a culturally competent assessment with women who have pelvic/sexual pain disorders and unwanted sexual experiences. Chapter 6 explains how to establish appropriate treatment goals and how to broaden treatment goals beyond the focus on pelvic/sexual pain. Chapter 7 reviews evidenced-based treatment techniques for treating women with pelvic/sexual pain and/or sexual trauma, which include graduated exposure therapy, psychoeducation, cognitive behavioral therapy, mindfulness skills, eye movement desensitization and reprocessing therapy, and behavioral sex therapy interventions. How to collaborate with other healthcare providers involved in the client's care and how and when to involve a partner in treatment are explored. Chapter 8 demonstrates the treatment of each case vignette. Chapter 9, the final chapter, identifies ideal conditions for termination, as well as factors that cause termination before a client may be ready.

## Important Takeaways

- Women's experiences of sexual trauma and pelvic/sexual pain have many parallels.
- Research is demonstrating the increased risk of developing a pelvic/sexual pain disorder for women who have experienced sexual and other psychological traumas and abuse.
- Institutional betrayal is common for women who have unwanted sexual experiences and can negatively impact recovery. Women with pelvic/sexual pain disorders may experience a form of institutional betrayal when seeking a diagnosis or treatment.

# References

Anderson, M., & Toor, S. (2020, August 25). *How social media users have discussed sexual harassment since #MeToo went viral.* Retrieved November 29, 2020, from www.pewresearch.org/fact-tank/2018/10/11/how-social-media-users-have-discussed-sexual-harassment-since-metoo-went-viral/

Black, M. C., Basile, K. C., Breiding, M. J., Smith, S. G., Walters, M. L., Merrick, M. T., Chen, J., & Stevens, M. R. (2011). *The national intimate partner and sexual violence survey (NISVS): 2010 summary report.* National Center for Injury Prevention and Control, Centers for Disease Control and Prevention. www.cdc.gov/violenceprevention/pdf/NISVS_Report2010-a.pdf

Cantor, D., Fisher, B., Chibnall, S., Harps, S., Townsend, R., Thomas, G., . . . Madden, K. (Revised January 17, 2020). *Report on the AAU campus climate survey on sexual assault and misconduct.* Prepared by Westat for the Association of American Universities.

Cohen, B., & Shenk, J. (Directors). (2020). *Athlete A* [Documentary]. Netflix.

Corsini-Munt, S., Bergeron, S., Rosen, N. O., Beaulieu, N., & Steben, M. (2016). A dyadic perspective on childhood maltreatment for women with provoked vestibulodynia and their partners: Associations with pain and sexual and psychosocial functioning. *The Journal of Sex Research,* 54(3), 308–318. doi:10.1080/00224499.2016.1158229

Del Pozo, O. (2019, November 26). *'Gender alert': Global protests denounce violence against women.* Retrieved December 01, 2020, from www.aljazeera.com/gallery/2019/11/26/gender-alert-global-protests-denounce-violence-against-women/

Di Caro, B. *#MeToo, #balancetonporc, #yotambien: Women around the world fight back at harassment.* Retrieved December 01, 2020, from www.weforum.org/agenda/2017/10/metoo-balancetonporc-yotambien-women-around-the-world-lash-out-at-harassment/

Duhart, D. T. (2001, December). *Violence in the Workplace, 1993–99.* US Department of Justice. Bureau of Justice Special Report: National Crime Victimization Survey. www.bjs.gov/content/pub/pdf/vw99.pdf

Evans, T. (2018, January 24). *Larry Nassar was sometimes arrogant, sometimes nervous, during only interview on sex abuse.* Retrieved December 02, 2020, from www.indystar.com/story/news/2018/01/23/larry-nassar-sometimes-confident-sometimes-arrogant-sometimes-nervous-during-only-interview-sex-abus/1054686001/

Freyd, J. J. (2021, November 2). *Institutional betrayal and institutional courage.* Retrieved November 13, 2021, from https://dynamic.uoregon.edu/jjf/institutionalbetrayal/

Get To Know Us: History & Inception. (2020, July 16). Retrieved November 29, 2020, from https://metoomvmt.org/get-to-know-us/history-inception/

Gibson, C. J., Li, Y., Inslicht, S. S., Seal, K. H., & Byers, A. L. (2018). Gender differences in cardiovascular risk related to diabetes and posttraumatic stress disorder. *The American Journal of Geriatric Psychiatry, 26*(12), 1268–1272. doi:10.1016/j.jagp.2018.09.012

Golshan, T. (2017, October 15). *Study finds 75 percent of workplace harassment victims experienced retaliation when they spoke up.* Retrieved December 03, 2020, from www.vox.com/identities/2017/10/15/16438750/weinstein-sexual-harassment-facts

Harlow, B. L., & Stewart, E. G. (2005). Adult-onset vulvodynia in relation to childhood violence victimization. *American Journal of Epidemiology, 161*(9), 871–880. doi:10.1093/aje/kwi108

Hauser, C., & Astor, M. (2018, January 25). *The Larry Nassar case: What happened and how the fallout is spreading.* Retrieved December 02, 2020, from www.nytimes.com/2018/01/25/sports/larry-nassar-gymnastics-abuse.html

Kearl, H. (2014). Unsafe and harassed in public spaces: A national street harassment report. *Stop Street Harassment.* www.stopstreetharassment.org/wp-content/uploads/2012/08/National-Street-Harassment-Report-November-29-20151.pdf

Khandker, M., Brady, S. S., Stewart, E. G., & Harlow, B. L. (2014). Is chronic stress during childhood associated with adult-onset vulvodynia? *Journal of Women's Health (Larchmont), 23*(8), 649–656.

Kozlowski, K. (2018, January 19). *What MSU knew: 14 were warned of Nassar abuse.* Retrieved December 03, 2020, from www.detroitnews.com/story/tech/2018/01/18/msu-president-told-nassar-complaint-2014/1042071001/

Landry, T., & Bergeron, S. (2011). Biopsychosocial factors associated with dyspareunia in a community sample of adolescent girls. *Archives of Sexual Behavior, 40*(5), 877–889. doi:10.1007/s10508-010-9637-9

Leclerc, B., Bergeron, S., Binik, Y. M., & Khalifé, S. (2010). History of sexual and physical abuse in women with dyspareunia: Association with pain, Psychosocial Adjustment, and sexual functioning. *The Journal of Sexual Medicine*, *7*(2), 971–980. https://doi.org/10.1111/j.1743-6109.2009.01581.x

McCoy Cohn, S., Cohn, P., & Zalace, A. (Producers), & McCoy Cohn, S. (Director). (2016). *Endo what?* [Documentary]. EndoWhat.org.

Miller, E., Beach, S. R., & Thurston, R. C. (2018). Addressing intimate partner violence and abuse of older or vulnerable adults in the health care setting – beyond screening. *JAMA Internal Medicine*, *178*(12), 1583. doi:10.1001/jamainternmed.2018.6523

#NousToutes. Retrieved December 01, 2020, from www.noustoutes.org/

Oppenheim, M. (2019, November 25). *Global protests demand end to violence against women*. Retrieved December 01, 2020, from www.independent.co.uk/news/world/politics/international-day-elimination-violence-against-women-protests-un-a9216996.html

Pflum, M. (2018, October 16). *A year ago, Alyssa Milano started a conversation about #MeToo. These women replied.* Retrieved November 29, 2020, from www.nbcnews.com/news/us-news/year-ago-alyssa-milano-started-conversation-about-metoo-these-women-n920246

Phillips, T. (2019, August 26). *Mexico's 'glitter revolution' targets violence against women*. Retrieved December 01, 2020, from www.theguardian.com/world/2019/aug/26/desperation-and-rage-mexican-women-take-to-streets-to-protest-unabated-sexual-violence-glitter-revolution

Rushworth, N. (2018, November 25). *#NousToutes: Tens of thousands protest violence against women in Paris*. Retrieved December 01, 2020, from www.france24.com/en/20181125-france-tens-thousands-protest-violence-against-women-paris

Smith, C. P., & Freyd, J. (2013, February). Dangerous safe havens: Institutional betrayal exacerbates sexual trauma. *The Journal of Traumatic Stress*, *26*, 119–124.

Stoltenborgh, M., Bakermans-Kranenburg, M. J., Alink, L. R., & van IJzendoorn, M. H. (2015). The prevalence of child maltreatment across the globe: Review of a series of meta-analyses. *Child Abuse Review*, *24*, 37–50.

Stone, M., & Vogelstein, R. (2019, March 07). *Celebrating #MeToo's global impact*. Retrieved November 29, 2020, from https://foreignpolicy.com/2019/03/07/metooglobalimpactinternationalwomens-day/

UNESCO. (2019, August 02). *Women make the news 2018*. Retrieved January 01, 2021, from https://en.unesco.org/womenmakenews

# 2

## COMMON PELVIC/SEXUAL PAIN DISORDERS

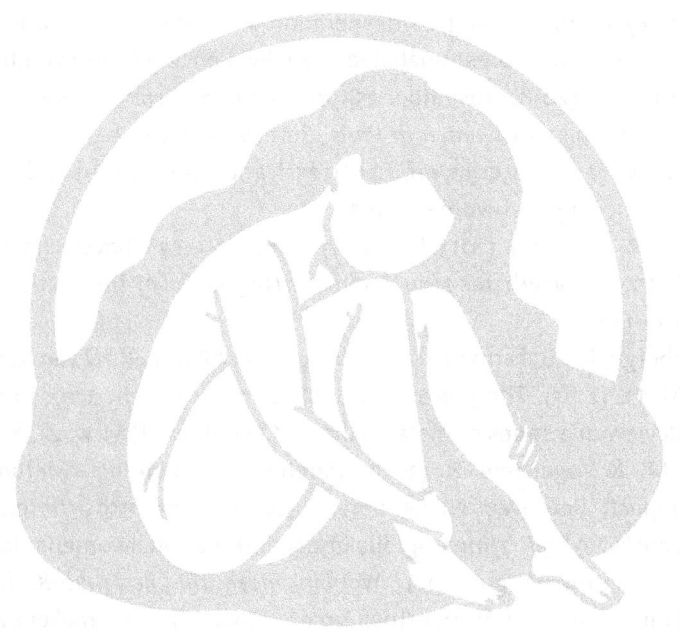

DOI: 10.4324/9781003168232-2

## Common Causes of Pelvic/Sexual Pain

Before we take a deeper dive into the connections between unwanted sexual experiences and pelvic/sexual pain disorders, we need to take a step back and learn about pelvic/sexual pain disorders because most mental health providers are not familiar with these conditions. There are some terms to be familiar with before diving deeper. *Dyspareunia* is a general term for "painful sex" and is commonly used in research studies to refer to a symptom caused by a range of pelvic/sexual conditions. Some healthcare providers may use the term *vaginismus* as a way to describe any kind of pelvic floor muscle dysfunction. However, when I use the term *vaginismus* during this book, I am referring to "lifelong vaginismus," meaning penetration of any kind (speculum, tampon, finger, penis) has never occurred.

Pelvic/sexual pain is quite common for women across their lifespan. One study found that 20% of sexually active adolescent girls reported vulvo-vaginal pain of more than 6 months' duration (Landry & Bergeron, 2011). The prevalence of genital pain among reproductive aged women in the general population ranges from 10% to 28% (Pukall et al., 2016a). Another study found the prevalence of painful sex to be 14% to 34% in younger women and 6.5% to 45% in older women (van Lankveld et al., 2010). Various disorders account for women's experiences of pelvic/sexual pain. In addition, it is common for women to have multiple disorders that are contributing to pelvic/sexual pain. Although not an exhaustive list, common causes of pelvic/sexual pain in women include:

1.  *Vulvodynia:* Vulvodynia is a chronic vulvar pain condition, which is estimated to be found in 8.3% of women (Reed et al., 2012). The most common presentation of vulvodynia is called provoked vestibulodynia, also called PVD (Harlow et al., 2001). Common symptoms include a burning, raw, sharp, stabbing, or tearing feeling at the entry of the vagina when pressure is applied to the area (Moyal-Barracco & Lynch, 2004; Henzell et al., 2017). Many of my clients with vulvodynia have experienced pain so significant that they find it difficult to wear pants and sometimes even underwear. Others may struggle with sitting for long periods of time. For those with high levels of vulvodynia pain, high distress is expected.

2.  *Pelvic floor dysfunction (PFD)*: PFD refers to a range of disorders that involve the pelvic floor muscles and other pelvic organs. Presentations of PFD may include urinary incontinence, fecal incontinence, and prolapse. The prevalence of PFD among women in the United States is estimated to be about 25% and increases as women age. Women with higher body mass indexes are also at greater risk of developing PFD (Wu et al., 2014). Most women have multiple factors or conditions that contribute to their PFD. While pain with sex is a common symptom for PFD, not all women with PFD experience pain with sex.

3.  *Vaginismus*: As previously stated, I am referring to lifelong vaginismus, or the experience of not being able to tolerate penetration of any form due to anxiety regarding penetration. It is estimated that the prevalence of vaginismus ranges from 0.4% to 6% (ter Kuile et al., 2015). However, meta-analyses suggest the rate varies based on geographic region and is about 6% to 31.6%. More religious or conservative cultures tend to report higher rates of vaginismus (McCool et al., 2016). This chapter further discusses the differences between vaginismus and other pelvic/sexual pain conditions. Although not always true, many of my clients with vaginismus have more conservative or sheltered upbringings. I commonly see obsessive-compulsive disorder and generalized anxiety disorder with vaginismus.

4.  *Endometriosis*: Endometriosis is a common reproductive disease in which endometrial tissue is found outside of the uterine cavity. Endometriosis adhesions grow on to various organs in the pelvis, causing chronic pain, painful intercourse, and infertility. Adhesions are commonly found on the outside of the uterus, fallopian tubes, uterosacral ligaments, peritoneum, bladder, ureters, vagina, and large and small bowel. However, endometriosis adhesions have been found as far as the diaphragm and lungs (Endometriosis Foundation of America, 2020). The disease is believed to impact 10% to 15% of all reproductive-age women and accounts for 70% of women that report chronic pelvic pain (Parasar et al., 2017). The presentation of endometriosis varies, and symptoms may be dependent on where the endometriosis has grown. Some women may have no physical symptoms and only become aware of a

possible endometriosis diagnosis when struggling with infertility. When women do experience symptoms, common symptoms include painful periods, spotting or bleeding in between periods, bleeding after intercourse, painful intercourse, pain with bowel movements, pain with urination, nausea and other gastrointestinal distress, general pelvic pain, fatigue, and nerve pain in the legs (Parasar et al., 2017; Endometriosis Foundation of America). The impact on sexual functioning for those with endometriosis is typically significant. An online study that surveyed 638 women with endometriosis in several countries, including the United States, found that 70% of women found sex unpleasant because of high levels of pain. Half of the respondents had pain that lasted 24 hours or more after sex (Witzeman et al., 2020). Many clients with endometriosis seek therapy because of the consequences of living with a chronic pelvic pain disorder, with relationship distress often being noted as a motivator to enter treatment.

5.  *Interstitial cystitis (IC)*: IC is also referred to as painful bladder syndrome. It is estimated that 2.7% to 6.53% of women have IC, with the range in estimate depending on the specificity and sensitivity of the definition used. Common symptoms include pelvic pain, bladder pressure and pain, and urinary urgency or frequency (Berry et al., 2011). Endometriosis and IC are commonly seen together (Paulson & Delgado, 2007). The impact on quality of life for those with IC can be significant, and many women have to plan their activities around access to bathrooms because of pain and urgency symptoms.

6.  *Physical trauma*: Physical trauma to the pelvic region, whether from surgery, an injury, or childbirth, can cause pelvic/sexual pain. At first attempt of penetrative sex postpartum, 85.7% of women reported pain with sex (McDonald et al., 2016). Another study found that 41% of women reported painful sex at three months postpartum and 22% at six months postpartum. The study also found that women with greater degrees of perineal trauma were much more likely to experience painful sex, as were women who needed the use of vacuum or forceps during delivery (Signorello et al., 2001). Women who had a cesarean delivery were also more likely to experience painful sex at six months postpartum compared

with women who had a vaginal delivery (McDonald et al., 2016). Childbirth with and without episiotomy, hysterectomy, and other genital procedures have also been linked to painful sex (Alligood-Percoco et al., 2016; Meana, 2012).

7.  *Hormonal changes:* Various hormonal changes across the lifespan put women at risk for experiencing pelvic/sexual pain. It is very common for women who are breastfeeding to experience painful sex due to lower levels of estrogen. In fact, women who breastfeed are four times more likely to experience painful sex than women who do not breastfeed postpartum (Signorello et al., 2001). Similarly, lower estrogen in postmenopausal women can cause changes in vaginal structure, elasticity, and lubrication, which can contribute to painful sex (Bergeron et al., 2015; van Lankveld et al., 2010). Treatment options for cancer include surgery, radiation therapy, chemotherapy, and medications that block hormones. These treatments may impact not only the physical structures of organs involved in penetrative sex but can also disrupt estrogen production, resulting in vaginal atrophy and difficulties with vaginal lubrication, contributing to pelvic/sexual pain (Mayo Clinic, 2020).

8.  *Uterine fibroids:* Uterine fibroids are benign tumors in the uterus that appear during women's reproductive ages. The estimated prevalence ranges between 5% and 21% of women, with higher incidence occurring in African American women. Common symptoms include heavy bleeding during periods, spotting in between periods, irregular periods, bladder pressure, pelvic pain, and pain during sex (Zimmermann et al., 2012). Similar to endometriosis, pain experienced with sex will depend on where the fibroids are located. Pain during or after intercourse can range from mild to quite severe (Fibroids and Sex: Fibroid Pain During Sex, n.d.).

9.  *Vulvar skin disorders:* A range of disorders can cause vulvar skin issues, including dermatitis or skin irritation caused by an allergy, lichen planus, lichen sclerosis, and Paget's disease. Women may also have psoriasis in the vulvar region or have skin irritation caused by infections, including chronic yeast infections or bacterial vaginosis. Common symptoms of vulvar skin disorders include itching, burning or stinging sensations, raw or dry skin, and skin lesions. It is important to note that the symptoms of the vulva might also

be indictors of a range of diseases, including gastrointestinal, blood, immune, and endocrine disorders. Vulvar skin conditions may cause pain with intercourse due to the skin irritation, skin thinning, and narrowing of the vaginal opening from scar tissue (Doyen et al., 2014).

10.    *Lack of education:* I believe it is important to include this cause of pelvic/ sexual pain because I have seen many clients whose pelvic/sexual pain was simply caused by engaging in penetrative sex before they were physically ready. Many women and their partners lack accurate information about the arousal process and how to know if their bodies are physically ready to engage in penetrative sex. If women attempt penetrative sex while not adequately aroused or lubricated, the result can be painful sex. I see this most often with clients who come from more conservative or more religious backgrounds. In fact, in traditional cultures of the Middle East and Asia, vaginismus, unconsummated marriage, and sexual pain are the most frequently reported female sexual problems (Heinemann et al., 2016). In the United States, women from all walks of life are lacking basic sexual knowledge. A poll commissioned by Intimina, a Swedish women's health company, surveyed 2,000 women in the United States and 25% of them did not know where their vagina was, 46% did not know where the cervix was, and 59% did not know where the uterus was. Only 10% of the women passed the anatomy quiz that asked them to name all of the parts of the female reproductive system (Sparks, 2020). The State of Period Report similarly found that 76% of respondents reported learning more about frog biology than the human female body in school (Broster, 2021). Therefore, do not assume that your even modern or liberal clients have received an adequate sexual education.

## Pelvic/Sexual Pain Disorders in the Case Vignettes
### Paula: Vulvodynia and Pelvic Floor Dysfunction

During her first pelvic exam at 17 years of age, Paula noted pain at the vaginal opening but believed this to be a normal part of a pelvic exam. She also recalled her doctor commenting at the exam that she would "get used to the discomfort." Later with her boyfriend from college, Paula noted that same burning pain at the entry of her vagina during any attempt of penetration, whether from a finger or penis. She explained she thought the symptoms would resolve but became worried when they persisted and prevented her from having intercourse. I referred her to a pelvic pain specialist, who diagnosed her with provoked vestibulodynia (a form of vulvodynia) and PFD.

### Violet: Endometriosis, Interstitial Cystitis, and Pelvic Floor Dysfunction

Periods had almost always been particularly painful and heavy for Violet, but her symptoms intensified and expanded over the years. Before receiving her diagnosis of endometriosis and PFD, Violet was not only experiencing disruptive periods but also significant fatigue, nausea, urinary frequency, bladder pain, significant back and hip pain, general pelvic pain, pain during sex, and sometimes spotting after sex. Violet was eventually referred to an endometriosis specialist, who performed a laparoscopic surgery confirming the suspected diagnosis. During the endometriosis laparoscopic surgery, a cystoscopy and hydrodistension of the bladder were performed due to Violet's urinary symptoms. These procedures confirmed the presence of IC. After the surgery, there was little follow-up or long-term treatment planning for either diagnosis. Upon entering therapy, I recommended Violet consult with a pelvic floor physical therapist. After a thorough evaluation, the pelvic floor physical therapist diagnosed PFD and noted significant myofascial restrictions.

### Rebecca: Suspected Pelvic Floor Dysfunction, Pudendal Nerve Entrapment, and/or Vulvodynia

Rebecca stated she did not have any pelvic/sexual pain issues until her skiing accident, but since then she had suffered for five years with various pelvic/sexual pain symptoms. The skiing accident resulted in a broken leg, dislocated shoulder, and a severe pelvic fracture. The pelvic fracture required surgery to repair, which was followed by a methicillin-resistant *Staphylococcus aureus* (MRSA) infection. Even after she had healed from the surgery and MRSA infection, her pain symptoms and physical limitations remained significant. Rebecca had received a range of diagnoses over the previous several years, including vulvodynia, PFD, pudendal nerve entrapment, fibromyalgia, somatization disorder, and so on, and had tried a range of evidenced-based medical treatments for these diagnoses with only mild improvements. Rebecca was referred to counseling by her pelvic floor physical therapist and OB/GYN specialist, who were puzzled by her lack of progress and suspected her psychological distress needed to be addressed.

### Siobhan: Lifelong Vaginismus

Technically, Siobhan had not experienced painful sex from any type of penetration because her anxiety prevented her from being able to even tolerate a pelvic exam. A previous OB/GYN had misdiagnosed Siobhan with vulvodynia after she reported pain during a "Q-tip" test, a common technique used to diagnose vulvodynia. In therapy, Siobhan later reflected that she was so panicked during the exam that she was not even sure if she had experienced pain and could not even recall the sensations she felt. She admitted being extremely fearful of the pain associated with intercourse and generally did not engage in much sexual activity beyond kissing and touching over her clothes with her husband. Siobhan did not experience pelvic pain symptoms in her daily life, like, for instance, from sitting for long periods of time. Upon meeting Siobhan, I suspected she had vaginismus and referred her to an OB/GYN who specialized in treating pelvic pain disorders. After meeting with the doctor, a diagnosis of vaginismus was confirmed. The OB/GYN specialist would teach Siobhan how to do dilator therapy and encouraged her to work with me on anxiety around dilator treatment and sexual experiences in general. The OB/GYN specialist suspected that Siobhan likely had some degree of PFD, but this could not be confirmed until she was physically and psychologically able to tolerate an internal pelvic exam.

### Noemi: Pelvic Floor Dysfunction and Vulvar Skin Irritation

After meeting with me for therapy and reporting painful sex with her husband since the birth of her first child, I referred Noemi to an OB/GYN specialist. The OB/GYN specialist diagnosed Noemi with

PFD and noted that her vulvar skin was very inflamed and irritated. Later in treatment, Noemi consulted with a pelvic floor physical therapist. The pelvic floor physical therapist also diagnosed Noemi with PFD and similarly noted how inflamed her vulvar skin was. She was referred to a vulvar skin specialist, who diagnosed her with an uncommon type of yeast infection and put her on a course of medication for several months to treat the infection. Estrogen cream was also prescribed because Noemi was on a low estrogen birth control pill.

## A Crash Course in the Pelvic Floor

Some of you are probably asking yourselves right now, "What the hell is a pelvic floor?" Most people have never heard of the pelvic floor or only do so when they experience an issue with their pelvic floor, leading me to one of my other points . . . how can you take care of a part of your body or seek treatment for a part of your body that no one told you existed? Louw et al. (2014) explain that pelvic/sexual pain patients often cannot see, or sometimes even name, the body part that is causing them pain, making it difficult to describe to others, including healthcare providers. This can increase frustration, fear, and anxiety, which in turn can increase the pain (p. 16).

For you to have a better understanding of female pelvic/sexual pain disorders and to provide your clients with basic psychoeducation about the pelvic floor, it is imperative to at least have some basic knowledge about the female pelvis (Figures 2.1 to 2.3 for an overview of the female pelvis). While therapists are not in a medical role, we are often one of the first professionals a client may discuss their pelvic/sexual pain symptoms with. Early psychoeducational conversations with clients who disclose pelvic/sexual pain, in addition to referring them to appropriate healthcare providers who can further assess and treat the physiological component, are crucial in a client's treatment. One of the easiest ways to explain the pelvic floor to clients is to have them imagine the pelvic floor as a bowl or hammock of both superficial and deep muscles. This bowl or hammock holds your bladder, uterus, vagina, and rectum and part of the bowel. The muscles serve as a "floor" for these organs and are the mechanism for constricting or closing the anus, vagina, and urethra (Raizada & Mittal, 2008).

# A crash course in the pelvic floor

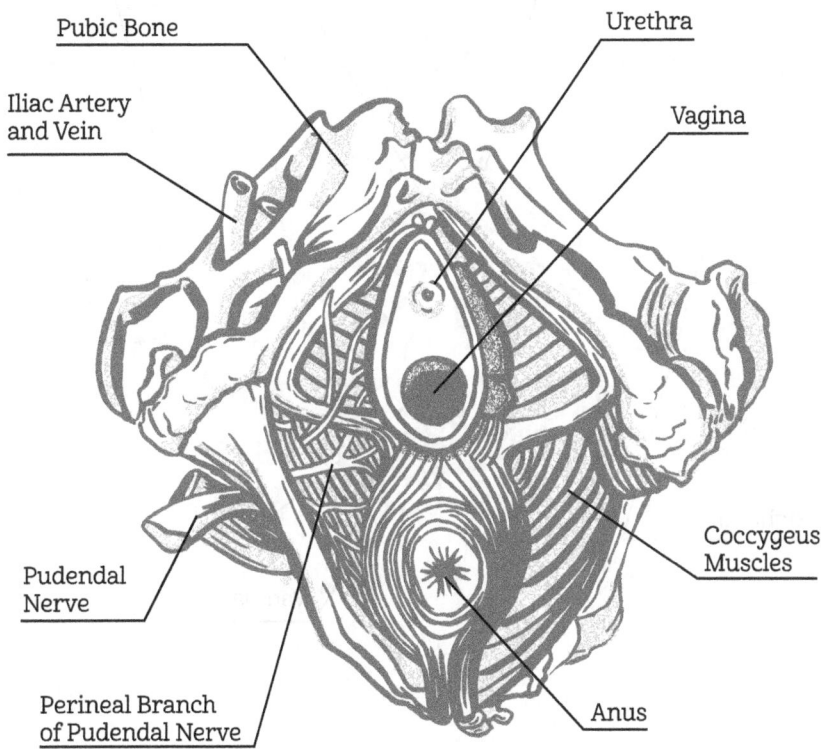

Pubic Bone

Urethra

Iliac Artery and Vein

Vagina

Coccygeus Muscles

Pudendal Nerve

Perineal Branch of Pudendal Nerve

Anus

## Basic Anatomy of the Pelvis

Because this muscle group is involved with so many different organ systems, a whole range of symptoms may present when PFD is occurring, including bladder pain, urinary frequency, urinary incontinence, difficulty emptying bladder, diarrhea, constipation, difficulty emptying

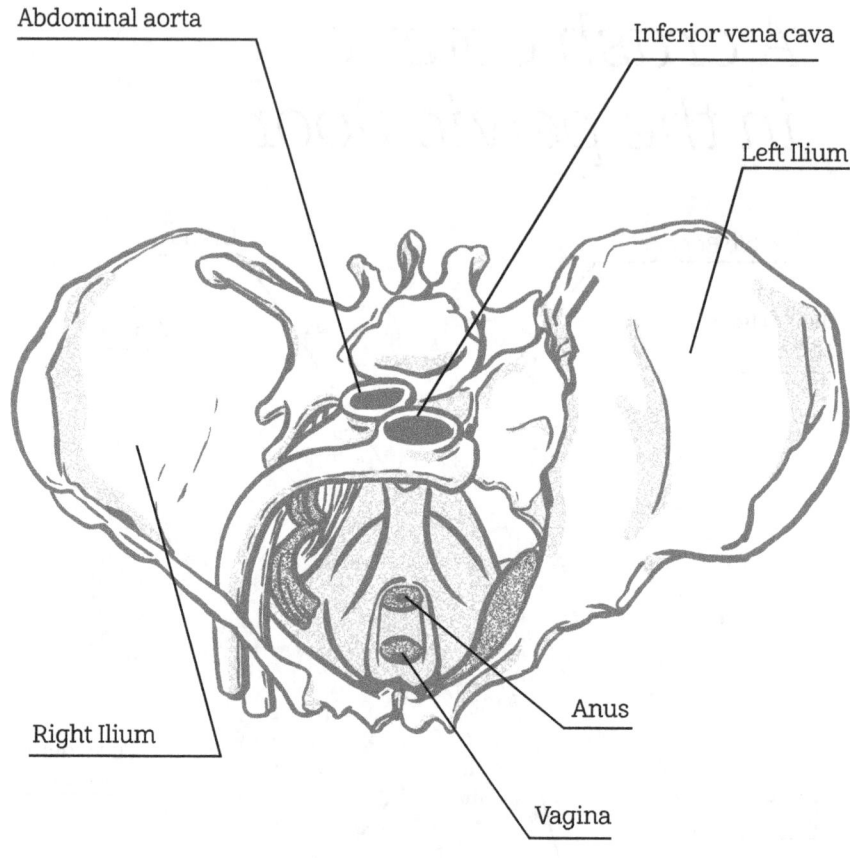

Abdominal aorta

Inferior vena cava

Left Ilium

Right Ilium

Anus

Vagina

## Superior View of the Pelvis

### (view from above)

bowels, low back pain, hip pain, tailbone pain, and painful intercourse (Pelvic Floor First, 2019). Often women with PFD believe they have irritable bowel syndrome (IBS) or chronic urinary infections, when the troubling symptoms are from PFDs. Note, however, that a woman may have IBS or chronic urinary infections, as well as PFD, which worsens

Iliac Crest

Vertebra Meets the Sacral base

Sacral Foramen
(houses S2 nerve root for pudendal nerve)

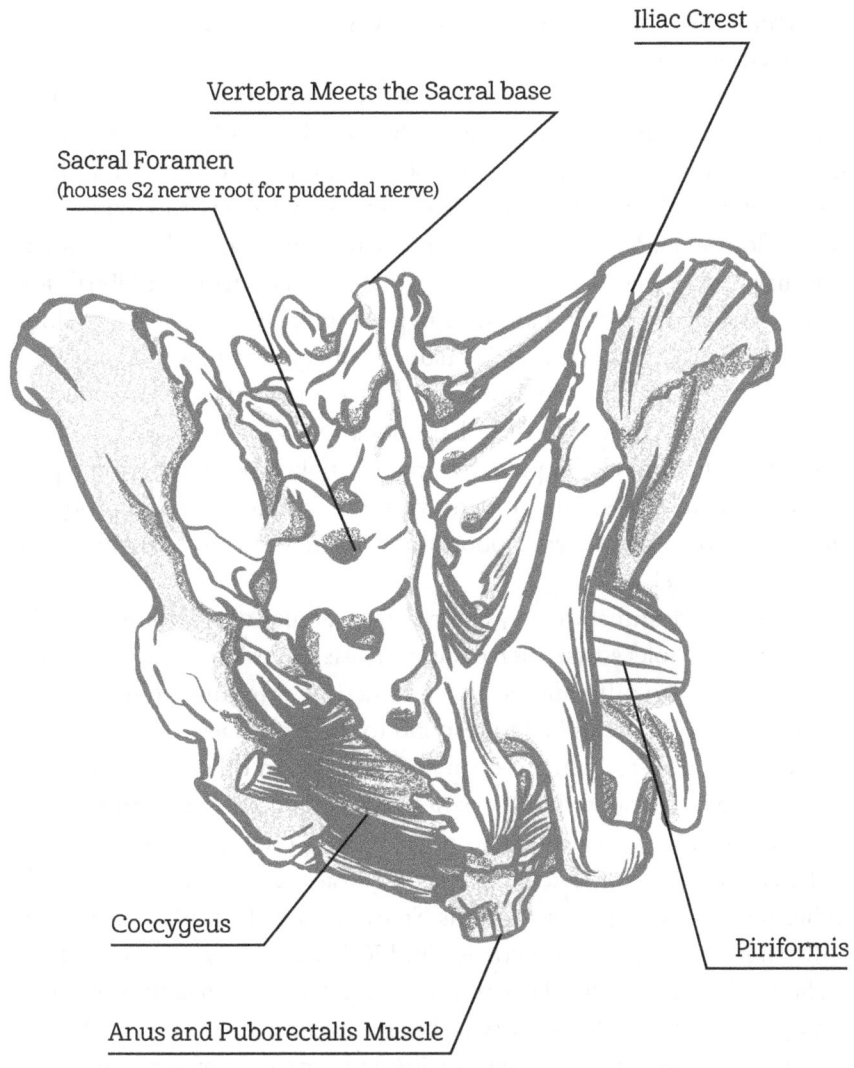

Coccygeus

Piriformis

Anus and Puborectalis Muscle

# Bony Landmarks and Relevant Soft Tissue
## of the Posterior Pelvis

the symptoms of these conditions. It is very common for clients to have PFD in addition to another pelvic/sexual pain disorder.

The pelvic floor muscles can sometimes be too weak or become hypertonic, which essentially means the muscles can become too tight. Stress and anxiety can contribute to the pelvic floor's becoming too tight. Pelvic/sexual pain conditions that have been associated with a hypertonic pelvic floor include vulvodynia, pudendal neuralgia, and IC. Women who have experienced perineal or vaginal tearing during childbirth are also at greater risk for developing a hypertonic pelvic floor (Pelvic Floor First, 2019). Using a hammock analogy, imagine yourself laying in a hammock. Ideally, the hammock should have nice give and respond to your shifting or moving in the hammock. Now imagine one or both sides of the hammock are pulled extremely tight (like a hypertonic pelvic floor). It would be difficult to move and would not be so comfortable either . . . now imagine your poor organs sitting in this extremely tight muscle hammock.

Pelvic floor dysfunction may contribute to a range of pelvic/sexual pain disorders. In Violet's case, her endometriosis adhesions had pulled her pelvic organs into different locations, sometimes binding them together. The pelvic floor muscles had to respond to these changes – overcompensating in some areas, while creating weaknesses in other areas. Because Violet was also living with daily pain from her endometriosis and IC, she carried her body in ways that were furthering these places of tightness and weakness in her pelvic floor. The PFD was contributing significantly to her pelvic/sexual pain symptoms. So even for a client like Violet, who will always live with endometriosis and IC because they are not curable, if she could improve her PFD and overall pelvic floor health, she could reduce her pain and the severity of her symptoms.

Various disorders, including pelvic/sexual pain disorders, can cause muscle pain, including in the pelvic floor. Sometimes this muscular pain is being driven by constricted fascia (Figures 2.4 and 2.5). Fascia is a type of connective tissue that is made up of layers of liquid called hyaluronan and is considered to be as sensitive as skin. This connective tissue surrounds our muscles, bones, nerves, organs, and blood vessels and helps with movement. Fascia restrictions occur when the fascia becomes thickened or too dry, causing muscle pain, joint stiffness, and muscle knots.

# Understanding the Fascia

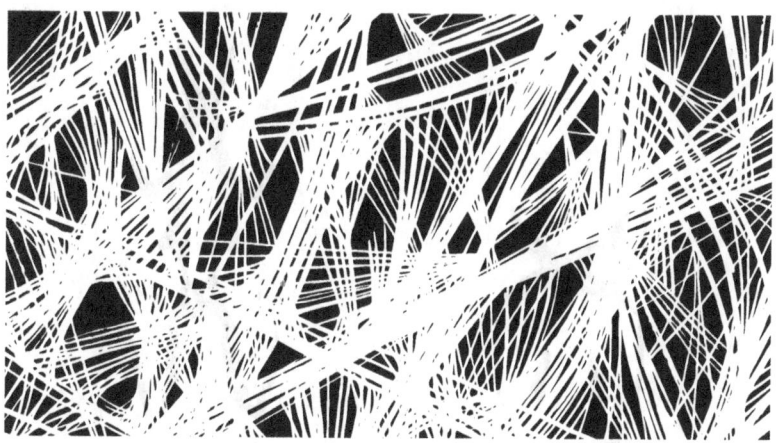

"Fascia is a thin covering of connective tissue that envelops organs, bones, nerves, muscles and blood vessels. It is like glue that keeps everything in place, keeping everything connected. It also has its own nerve network. When the central nervous system is ramped up or excitable, the fascia can reflect this and become very tight. When fascia is healthy, it is mobile and can glide and twist and bend. But inflammation and trauma can cause fascia to tighten, which then contributes to pain. For many individuals, modalities like pelvic floor physical therapy address fascial contribution to pain in addition to specific muscles and other connective tissue. Releasing fascial constrictions can be very helpful in treating pain."

**- Stephanie Muntzer, MPT, PYT, RYT 200, CPI,**
Founder and Owner of Blend Physical Therapy

# How the Fascia Interconnects

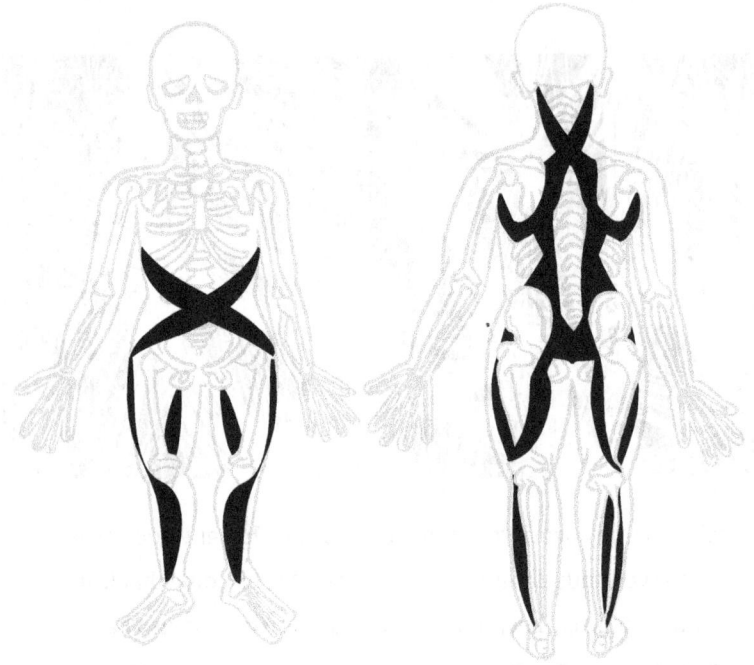

"When we are treating connective tissue dysfunction in our patients, we often see patterns of restriction and tightness that aren't specific to one body part or area. Essentially everything is connected. In the past we treated certain body parts individually, but the fascia is helping us to understand how one body part is connected to another. An example of this is a restriction in the shoulder contributing to dysfunction and pain in the pelvis."

**- Stephanie Muntzer, MPT, PYT, RYT 200, CPI,**
Founder and Owner of Blend Physical Therapy

This can be triggered by stress, limited mobility, repetitive movement, or physical trauma (Johns Hopkins Medicine, 2020).

Because there are so many different factors as to what could be causing pelvic/sexual pain and our clients often lack knowledge about the pelvic floor, it can be difficult for clients to put into words their pelvic/sexual pain experiences. It is important for clinicians to be able to have a basic conversation about the location of the pain, the type of pain, and triggers for the pain. Sometimes clients cannot specifically identify where the pain is. I ask clients to think about three main areas of their pelvis where the pain might be: (1) the vulva (external genitalia), (2) vestibule (the entrance to the vagina), and (3) deep pelvic pain. Pelvic/sexual pain sensations range from mild to severe and could include any of the following descriptive words: dull, achy, raw, stabbing, burning, itching, sharp, throbbing, shooting, stinging, or nagging (Figure 2.6).

When clients struggle with words to describe the pain, I encourage them to create an image for me: If your pain could be a shape, what would it be? A size? If it could have a temperature? A color? A sound? As a clinician, you also need to know when the pain is occurring or what types of pain are occurring with certain activities. For instance, some women may experience a very distinct sharp or burning pain upon penetration attempts at the vestibule, but otherwise their pain is dull or nagging. Just as it is important to know the triggers for the pain, it is also important to ask clients about what reduces or relieves the pain.

Facilitating conversations about the pain is very important. First, it is a way to establish an alliance with the client, who mostly likely has been dismissed about her pain by other professionals. Listening and wanting to understand the details and nuances about the client's pelvic/sexual pain conveys not only that you take the matter seriously but also that her pelvic/sexual pain is not some unsolvable or untreatable medical mystery (a message that sadly many have been given). The conversation can also help clients to better understand their pain and gives language or imagery to something that likely has been difficult to communicate about. In addition, it serves as practice for talking with healthcare providers about their pelvic/sexual pain. Being able to communicate clearly and directly about pelvic/sexual pain is important in helping healthcare providers to diagnose and treat these complex issues. As therapists, we

# Pain Chart

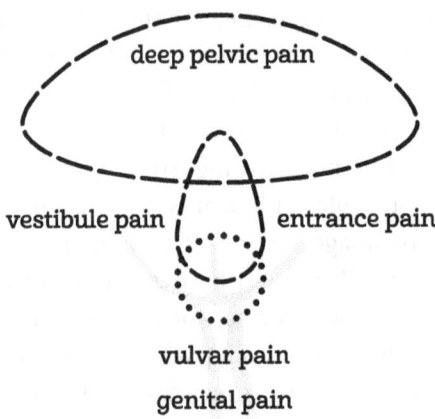

deep pelvic pain

vestibule pain        entrance pain

vulvar pain

genital pain

## Type of pain:

burning    stinging    stabbing    throbbing    itching

dull    sharp    achy    heavy    nagging    shooting

## When is the pain occurring?

All of the time? With only certain activities?

At certain points in your cycle?

do not diagnosis the pain beyond the DSM-V diagnosis of genito-pelvic pain/penetration disorder (GPPPD). However, we need to understand the symptoms, including the details about the pelvic/sexual pain, to make the most appropriate referrals to medical specialists, and to understand the greater impact of the pelvic/sexual pain condition on the client's daily life.

## Important Changes in the *DSM-V* Regarding Diagnosing Pelvic/Sexual Pain

The DSM-V (2013) merged the previous diagnoses of vaginismus and dyspareunia into a singular diagnosis, GPPPD (APA, 2013). To be diagnosed with GPPPD, a client must experience one or more of the following: (1) difficulty with vaginal penetration during intercourse, (2) experiencing vaginal pain during intercourse, (3) fear or anxiety related to vaginal penetration or pain during penetration, or (4) tightening of pelvic floors muscles prior to or during intercourse. The subtypes include lifelong versus acquired. However, the DSM-V criteria for lifelong is based on when a person first becomes sexually active. The recent DSM-V changes reflect the latest research, which indicates the overlap in symptoms and presentation of dyspareunia and vaginismus, as well as research indicating that the idea of vaginal spasm is not adequate in the diagnosis of vaginismus (Cherner & Reissing, 2013).

Over the past 15 to 20 years, various studies have demonstrated the comorbidity of vaginismus and dyspareunia. Van Lankveld et al. (1995) found that when examining predictors of vaginismus, dyspareunia, and mixed sexual pain disorder in a retrospective study, no differences were found among these groups. Kruiff et al. (2000) found no significant differences between patients with vaginismus or dyspareunia in their reported pain levels during intercourse or attempted intercourse or in their ability to insert a finger or to complete a gynecological exam. The only difference found among the groups was that the patients with vaginismus were more likely to report intercourse to be impossible.

In tune with the new diagnostic criteria, GPPPD does not require a patient to have experienced vaginal spasm. Historically, the idea and role of the muscle spasm were important in the diagnosis of vaginismus. However, there was never a consensus regarding the definition of spasm nor a consensus about distinguishing different types of muscle contractions or cramps (Reissing et al., 2004; ter Kuile & Reissing, 2014). Even without a clear definition of spasm, fewer than a third of women with vaginismus presented with a vaginal/pelvic spasm during gynecological exams (Reissing et al., 2004). Additional research has found that the vaginal spasm is invalid and unreliable in the diagnosis of vaginismus (Cherner & Reissing, 2013; Lahaie et al., 2010; ter Kuile & Reissing, 2014).

## Lifelong Vaginismus Conceptualized as a Specific Phobia

The previously discussed research findings are important in identifying the similarities between dyspareunia and acquired vaginismus. However, the recent changes within the DSM-V (2013) overlook the experiences and difficulties of women with lifelong vaginismus (Reissing et al., 2014). Because of these changes, some argue that the diagnosis of GPPPD does not reflect the complex symptomatology of lifelong vaginismus (Reissing et al., 2014). It is important as clinicians to understand the differences between vaginismus and GPPPD because there are treatment implications.

The research on lifelong vaginismus supports its discrepancy from GPPPD. Women with lifelong vaginismus differed in their manifestation of anxiety and fear during pelvic examinations compared with women with dyspareunia. They also expressed high levels of anxiety and fear, preventing the pelvic examinations (ter Kuile et al., 2009). The fear leads to avoidance of any experiences that could result in vaginal penetration and in turn eliminates opportunities that could challenge the cognitive distortions that maintain the fear and avoidance (ter Kuile et al., 2009, p. 150; Reissing et al., 2014). This avoidance negatively reinforces the fear-avoidance cycle of vaginismus, similar to that of a specific phobia (Cherner & Reissing, 2013, p. 1612). According to ter Kuile and Reissing (2014) the fear-avoidance model of vaginismus developed by Vlaeyen and Linton (2000) explains how vaginal penetration problems are exacerbated in women who already have anxiety and/or pain when attempting intercourse, thus leading to a cyclical pattern of pain and avoidance.

Van Lankveld's et al. (1995) conceptualized lifelong vaginismus as a specific phobia. When examining the cognitions of women with lifelong vaginismus compared with those with dyspareunia, several important differences emerged. The fear of pain was the primary reason women with vaginismus reported to avoid intercourse (Lahaie et al., 2010). "Women with lifelong vaginismus report significantly more negative cognitions related to vaginal penetration and have higher pain catastrophizing cognitions when compared to women without sexual pain and women with dyspareunia" (Reissing et al., 2014, p. 1211). These women also reported "significantly more causal attributions related to fears of pain, injury, intimacy, and loss of control, and negative images of the body and their own genitals and penis, disgust about intercourse" (Cherner & Reissing, 2013, p. 1606). A study by Borg et al. (2014) used magnetic resonance imaging to determine if women with vaginismus demonstrate similar brain responses towards intercourse and images intended to disgust. While the women with vaginismus reported the intercourse stimuli as more disgusting than women without sexual pain or vaginismus, the actual brain responses did not differ between these two groups. The research team hypothesized that perhaps the findings point to conflict regarding the drive to procreate and experience pleasure versus feeling contaminated and disgusted about penetration.

In many ways, Siobhan fit the profile of a typical lifelong vaginismus case. She initially reported experiencing severe pain during her first OB/GYN pelvic exam but eventually in therapy realized she was not even sure if the doctor was able to physically touch her other than with a Q-tip. When the Q-tip test was performed, she reported the pain to be severe but was so panicked and possibly dissociated during the experience. She acknowledged this may have interfered with her body's interpretation of sensation. As Siobhan later reflected in therapy after accomplishing insertion with dilator number one, "I think before my body was sending me pain signals, but it was not because I was in pain. It was because I was so anxious, and my body was telling me to get out of there, get away from the threat, the thing that was giving me anxiety [the pelvic exam]." During the assessment, it was clear Siobhan had very negative cognitions about sex, her body, and her husband's body. She reported believing intercourse would not be possible and likened the pain to "getting stabbed with a sword." She had never looked at her own genitalia and had not allowed her husband to see her naked from the waist down. So, unlike other women with pelvic/sexual pain disorders, for women with lifelong vaginismus like Siobhan, it is the fear of the pain, usually not experienced pain, that drives anxiety and avoidance of penetration.

## Trauma and the Pelvis

While many therapists acknowledge the mind and body connection, most lack specific knowledge regarding this connection when it comes to the pelvis. As I noted in Chapter 1, several studies have noted the increased risk of developing a pelvic/sexual pain disorder among adolescent girls and adult women who have had traumatic life experiences, including sexual trauma (Landry & Bergeron, 2011; Harlow & Stewart, 2005; Corsini-Munt et al., 2016; Khandker et al., 2014). Living in a traumatized state or under chronic stress causes changes in the body, which could contribute to a pelvic/sexual pain disorder. In fact, research indicates that posttraumatic stress disorder and other chronic pain conditions may increase the risk of developing vulvodynia (Reed et al., 2012).

One study used surface Electric and Magnetic Field (EMF) sensors on women with and without vaginismus and then had them view sexually threatening films. Both groups of women showed increased muscle activity when watching the sexually threatening films. This led the researchers to conclude that increased pelvic muscle tension and contractions may be used by all women as a protective mechanism in response to a threat (van der Velde et al., 2001). This is a very interesting and important finding, as it calls in to question what happens for women who are stuck in a trauma state, physically responding to most stimuli as if it were still a danger or threat. For women who are living under continuous threat to their wellbeing or safety or under a chronic state of stress, it is possible that their pelvic floor muscles tense in response, contributing to or causing pelvic/sexual pain.

As Louw et al. (2014) explain in *Why Pelvic Pain Hurts: Neuroscience Education for Patients with Pelvic Pain*:

> Even though there may be specific causes for pelvic pain, they all share common features in regard to how the pain develops and persists. In medicine, we often overcomplicate pain. Pain is 100% produced by the brain. Pain is produced when the brain perceives there is a threat and protection is needed. . . . If there's little threat, pain is not produced. If the brain believes there's a credible threat, pain is produced.
>
> (p. 20)

This explanation resonated with Noemi, who had both sexual trauma and recent medical trauma. Once she started experiencing painful intercourse after her first baby, she stated whenever she thought her husband might be interested in sex, she treated him "as if he were a threat." She found herself lashing out at him or withdrawing when he made attempts to initiate sex, as she was attempting to avoid not only the pain but also the traumatic memories. After reading this book during counseling, Rebecca finally had a possible explanation for why her severe chronic pelvic pain had persisted long after her accident, surgery, and recovery from infection. She questioned whether perhaps her nervous system was stuck in responding as if it were constantly under threat of attack and therefore continued to produce pain despite receiving appropriate medical treatment for her suspected diagnoses.

Siobhan also resonated with this explanation and felt as though it explained why perhaps she "felt pain, even though I do not even think the doctor touched me – at least not more than a second or two." Her fear about the pain associated with penetration kept her body on alert and anticipating pain anytime there was a possible threat (a tampon, a doctor attempting an exam, her husband attempting intercourse). Siobhan began to listen to her body when it produced pain sensations, explaining that "perhaps it's just trying to send me a message." It is helpful to explain to clients that pain is simply one way our body communicates. If they can start to view pain as a method of dialogue, pain has less of a negative association.

Another component to painful intercourse that pain interferes with the body's sexual response cycle, therefore increasing the likelihood of experiencing pain with sex. If sex is consciously or unconsciously viewed as a threat, the pelvic floor muscles tighten and pain signals fire, thereby disrupting vasocongestion and lubrication. A study on women with endometriosis highlighted this pattern. The study found that for women with endometriosis, fear and the anticipation of pain disrupt the sexual response cycle, which can in turn create low sexual desire and difficulties with lubrication (Norinho et al., 2020). Difficulties with desire, arousal, and lubrication can contribute to painful intercourse.

Earlier we learned how stress can cause the fascia to tighten, causing muscle pain and stiffness (Johns Hopkins Medicine, 2020). Other research has looked at the impact of stress on the endometriosis growths.

When researchers in Japan studied the relationship between mental stress and endometriosis using mice, they found that mental stress might encourage the growth of endometriosis lesions and cause an inflammatory reaction on the tissue surrounding the uterus. Based on the results in the mice, they believe reducing stress or avoiding stress can prevent the progression of endometriosis (Kawakita et al., 2020). So even when a pelvic/sexual pain condition like endometriosis already exists, a client now living in a traumatized state or living with chronic stress is likely to experience increased pain and other disruptive symptoms because of the impact of the stress.

## The Impact of Pelvic/Sexual Pain Disorders on Quality of Life

When most people think of pelvic/sexual pain disorders, they most commonly think of the impact on sexual functioning or the ability to have pain-free sex. However, research shows the impact reaches beyond painful intercourse and distress over sexual functioning. Painful intercourse does seem to be an indicator of the overall impact of the condition on quality of life. For instance, Dutch researchers found that in women with endometriosis, painful intercourse, more severe period pain, worse health-related quality of life, and unemployment were associated with worse quality of life (Poll et al., 2020). A study of Spanish women who had endometriosis found their mean Female Sexual Function Inventory (FSFI) score to be 22.5, well below the cutoff score of 26.5 for normal sexual function. While sexual and pelvic pain influenced the sexual functioning of the women with endometriosis, the researchers also found that the strongest predictive factors of poor sexual functioning were deep endometriosis, depression level, age, and unemployment (González-Mesa et al., 2021). Another study of women ages 18 to 25 years of age found that women with endometriosis experienced painful intercourse twice as often as the women without endometriosis. Respondents who reported having painful intercourse endorsed lower physical and mental health quality of life scores, with the impact being stronger in women with endometriosis. The authors concluded that assessing painful intercourse should be a part of reproductive healthcare because it has such significant impacts on social functioning and mental and physical health (Schneider et al., 2020). These studies highlight the interplay of sexual functioning and other quality of life measures.

Beyond sex, it is crucial to understand the broad impact pelvic/sexual pain disorders have on women's quality of life, including their financial stability and workforce participation. For endometriosis alone, the estimated yearly financial burden is $69.4 billion, which includes direct healthcare costs and loss of productivity. It should be noted that these estimates were based on statistics from 2010, so the estimate to date is likely much higher (Soliman et al., 2018). Similarly, a Canadian study surveyed 30,000 women and found that the 2,000 women who reported an endometriosis diagnosis experienced fatigue and productivity impairment significantly greater than women who did not report an endometriosis diagnosis (Soliman et al., 2021). A study conducted in Australia on the social and economic impact of endometriosis on women's lives found that women felt a lack of understanding and support from friends and family. Of the 200 participants, 86% reported a negative impact on leisure activities, including being able to attend social events, due to physical symptoms of endometriosis. More than 40% of respondents reported exhausting their sick leave or unpaid leave because of their endometriosis (Mastrangelo & Turnbull, 2021). Fatigue and productivity impairment from endometriosis directly impacts women's ability to participate in leisure and social activities, as well as and school and work. The negative impact to school and work participation, however, directly contributes to financially instability over time, creating an additional barrier to receiving adequate treatment.

Researchers in Portugal conducted a review of 10 articles that highlighted the experiences of 582 women with endometriosis and 411 partners of women with endometriosis. The researchers found many impacts of the disease beyond pain with sex. The study noted that depression and anxiety related to endometriosis created issues in romantic relationships, work, and school. Many women also reported feeling distress about infertility and had concerns about the impact of future surgeries. The study also found that because clinics do not offer women with endometriosis or their partners couples or sex therapy, many couples are left with little support and have significant concerns about their futures (Norinho et al., 2020).

The impacts of endometriosis have been found to negatively impact women's mental health. A BBC study that surveyed 13,500 women with endometriosis found that half of them reported suicidal thoughts, mostly due to the lack of support around diagnosing and treating the disease. The women also reported significant negative impacts to their relationships, careers, and education (Bevan, 2019). A 2020 study (Estes et al., 2020) found that women with endometriosis, especially those who reported painful periods, painful sex, and pelvic pain, reported significantly higher rates of anxiety, depression, and self-harm behaviors. Researchers in Brazil found that 90% of women with bowel endometriosis had depression, anxiety, or both (Ribeiro et al., 2021). In addition to experiencing mental health issues, a recent study found that women with endometriosis are at a four-time greater risk of chronic opioid use compared with women without endometriosis (Chiuve et al., 2021).

Consistent with the broad and negative impact endometriosis has on women's lives, similar findings have been noted in regard to other pelvic/sexual pain conditions. For instance, the quality of life for people with IC was ranked lower than for those undergoing chronic dialysis for renal failure (Hanno, 2002). Another study looking at the symptoms of uterine fibroids and the impact of the disease found that 53.7% of women reported the condition had negatively impacted their lives in the previous 12 months. Of the respondents, 42.9% said their sex lives were negatively impacted, 27.7% said their work performance was negatively impacted, and 27.2% said their relationships and interactions with family had been negatively impacted (Zimmermann et al., 2012).

Like most women with pelvic/sexual pain disorders, Paula, Violet, Rebecca, and Noemi's ability to have pain-free and pleasurable sex had been impacted. For Paula, she worried about whether her boyfriend would leave and find a "normal girl." While Noemi felt secure in her marriage despite their recent conflicts, she did believe the lack of sexual connection was negatively impacting their emotional intimacy and overall happiness. Violet explained that dating seemed daunting, and she often struggled with when was appropriate to disclose about her endometriosis, IC, and sexual difficulties. "Who would sign up for that?" Violet often lamented and expressed being particularly worried about her infertility. Rebecca, who had enjoyed an active and healthy sex life for most of her marriage, knew the lack of sexual connection since her accident had contributed the current marital distress. While Siobhan was not having penetrative sex, she worried about whether her marriage would survive if it remained unconsummated.

Violet's endometriosis had significantly impacted her education and career path. She had always prioritized school but nearly every month would lose several days to her endometriosis symptoms. It also prevented her from being able to engage in other activities that would have strengthened her resume like becoming a research assistant or taking on more teaching opportunities. In Rebecca's case, the severity of her pelvic pain symptoms caused her to leave her job as a paralegal. Although her family was not hurting from the loss of income, the inability to work and contribute financially had negatively impacted her self-confidence. Siobhan, Violet, Paula, and Noemi all struggled with carving out the time needed for regular treatment, including physical therapy, appointments with specialists, engaging in physical therapy or other exercises at home, and counseling. Often the amount of time needed to effectively treat and initially manage a pelvic/sexual pain condition adds up to several hours each week. This time demand could obviously negatively impact education, career, and long-term financial security.

## Important Takeaways

- Causes of pelvic/sexual pain commonly include vulvodynia, PFD, vaginismus, endometriosis, IC, physical trauma, hormonal changes, uterine fibroids, vulvar skin disorders, and lack of education.
- The *DSM-V* merged the previous diagnoses of vaginismus and dyspareunia into a singular diagnosis of GPPPD due to an overlap in the symptoms and presentations of these disorders.
- Lifelong vaginismus presents differently from other pelvic/sexual pain disorders, and some experts in the field argue it should be conceptualized as a phobia.
- Research shows that chronic stress or living in a "trauma state" can exacerbate pelvic/sexual pain conditions.
- Pelvic/sexual pain disorders not only negatively impact women's sexual functioning, but research has shown they also negatively impact overall quality of life, relationships with others, and financial stability.

# References

Alligood-Percoco, N. R., Kjerulff, K. H., & Repke, J. T. (2016). Risk factors for dyspareunia after first childbirth. *Obstetrics and Gynecology, 128*(3), 512.

American Psychiatric Association. (2013). Sexual dysfunctions. In *Diagnostic and statistical manual of mental disorders* (5th ed.). http://dsm.psychia tryonline.org.proxy1.lib.tju.edu/doi/full/10.1176/appi.books.9780890 425596.dsm13#CIHCHEFI

Bergeron, S., Corsini-Munt, S., Aerts, L., Rancourt, K., & Rosen, N. O. (2015). Female sexual pain disorders: A review of the literature on etiology and treatment. *Current Sexual Health Reports, 7*(3), 159–169.

Berry, S. H., Elliott, M. N., Suttorp, M., Bogart, L. M., Stoto, M. A., Eggers, P., . . . Clemens, J. Q. (2011). Prevalence of symptoms of bladder pain syndrome/interstitial cystitis among adult females in the United States. *Journal of Urology, 186*(2), 540–544. doi:10.1016/j.juro.2011.03.132

Bevan, G. (2019, October 06). *Endometriosis: Thousands share devastating impact of condition.* Retrieved December 28, 2020, from www.bbc. com/news/health-49897873

Borg, C., Georgiadis, J. R., Renken, R. J., Spoelstra, S. K., Weijmar Schultz, W., & de Jong, P. J. (2014). Brain processing of visual stimuli representing sexual penetration versus core and animal-reminder disgust in women with lifelong vaginismus. *PLoS ONE, 9*(1). https://doi.org/10.1371/journal. pone.0084882

Broster, A. (2021, May 31). *76% of students learn more about the biology of frogs than the human female BODY, according to study.* Retrieved June 21, 2021, from www.forbes.com/sites/alicebroster/2021/05/31/76- of-students-learn-more-about-the-biology-of-frogs-than-the-human- female-body-according-to-study/?sh=679438795ddd

Cancer treatment for women: Possible sexual side effects. (2020, June 06). Retrieved December 20, 2020, from www.mayoclinic.org/ diseases-conditions/cancer/in-depth/cancer-treatment/art-20047214

Cherner, R., & Reissing, E. (2013). A comparative study of sexual function, behavior, and cognitions of women with lifelong vaginismus. *Archives of Sexual Behavior, 42*, 1605–1614. doi:10.1007/s10508-013-0111-3

Chiuve, S. E., Kilpatrick, R. D., Hornstein, M. D., Petruski-Ivleva, N., Wegrzyn, L. R., Dabrowski, E. C., . . . Bateman, B. T. (2021). Chronic opioid use and complication risks in women with endometriosis: A cohort study in us administrative claims. *Pharmacoepidemiology and Drug Safety.* doi:10.1002/pds.5209

Corsini-Munt, S., Bergeron, S., Rosen, N. O., Beaulieu, N., & Steben, M. (2016). A dyadic perspective on childhood maltreatment for women with provoked vestibulodynia and their partners: Associations with pain and sexual and psychosocial functioning. *The Journal of Sex Research, 54*(3), 308–318. doi:10.1080/00224499.2016.1158229

Doyen, J., Demoulin, S., Delbecque, K., Goffin, F., Kridelka, F., & Delvenne, P. (2014). Vulvar skin disorders throughout lifetime: About some representative dermatoses. *BioMed Research International, 2014*, 1–6. doi:10.1155/2014/595286

Endometriosis, A-Z. (2020, July 30). *The endometriosis foundation of America.* Retrieved on December 19, 2020, from www.endofound.org/endometriosis-a-to-z

Estes, S. J., Huisingh, C. E., Chiuve, S. E., Petruski-Ivleva, N., & Missmer, S. A. (2020). Depression, anxiety, and self-directed violence in women with endometriosis: A retrospective matched-cohort study. *American Journal of Epidemiology, 190*(5), 843–852. doi:10.1093/aje/kwaa249

Fibroids and Sex: Fibroid Pain During Sex. (n.d.). Retrieved December 19, 2020, from www.usafibroidcenters.com/uterine-fibroid-symptoms/pain-during-sex/

González-Mesa, E., Moya-Bejarano, D., Butrón-Hinojo, C. A., Marín-Sánchez, P., Blasco-Alonso, M., Jimenez-López, J. S., Villegas-Muñoz, E., & Lubián-López, D. M. (2021). Correlates of sexual function in a sample of Spanish women with endometriosis. *Journal of Clinical Medicine, 10*(21), 4957. https://doi.org/10.3390/jcm10214957

Hanno, P. M. (2002). Interstitial cystitis-epidemiology, diagnostic criteria, clinical markers. *Reviews in Urology, 4*(Suppl 1), S3–S8.

Harlow, B. L., & Stewart, E. G. (2005). Adult-onset vulvodynia in relation to childhood violence victimization. *American Journal of Epidemiology, 161*(9), 871–880. doi:10.1093/aje/kwi108

Harlow, B. L., Wise, L. A., & Stewart, E. G. (2001). Prevalence and predictors of chronic lower genital tract discomfort. *American Journal of Obstetrics and Gynecology, 185*, 545–550. dio:10.1067/mob.2001.116748

Heinemann, J., Atallah, S., & Rosenbaum, T. (2016). The impact of culture and ethnicity on sexuality and sexual function. *Current Sexual Health Reports, 8*(3), 144–150.

Henzell, H., Berzins, K., & Langford, J. P. (2017). Provoked vestibulodynia: Current perspectives. *International Journal of Women's Health, 9,* 631–642. dio:10.2147/IJWH.S113416

Johns Hopkins Medicine. (2020). *Muscle pain: It may actually be your fascia.* Retrieved December 26, 2020, from www.hopkinsmedicine.org/health/wellness-and-prevention/muscle-pain-it-may-actually-be-your-fascia

Kawakita, T., Kato, T., Iwasa, T., Erdenebayar, O., Kadota, Y., Kasai, K., . . . Irahara, M. (2020). Mental stress promotes the proliferation of endometriotic lesions in mice. *Cytokine, 135,* 155222. doi:10.1016/j.cyto.2020.155222

Khandker, M., Brady, S. S., Stewart, E. G., & Harlow, B. L. (2014). Is chronic stress during childhood associated with adult-onset vulvodynia? *Journal of Women's Health (Larchmont), 23*(8), 649–656.

Kruiff, M., ter Kuile, M., Weijenborg, P., & Van Lankveld, J. J. (2000). Vaginismus and dyspareunia: Is there a difference in clinical presentation? *Journal of Psychosomatic Obstetrics & Gynecology, 21,* 149–155. doi:10.3109/01674820009075622

Lahaie, M., Boyer, S., Amsel, R., Khalifé, S., & Binik, Y. (2010). Vaginismus: A review of the literature on the classification/diagnosis, etiology and treatment. *Women's Health, 6,* 705–719. doi:10.2217/whe.10.46

Landry, T., & Bergeron, S. (2011). Biopsychosocial factors associated with dyspareunia in a community sample of adolescent girls. *Archives of Sexual Behavior, 40*(5), 877–889.

Louw, A., Hilton, S., & Vandyken, C. (2014). *Why pelvic pain hurts: Neuroscience education for patients with pelvic pain.* International Spine and Pain Institute.

Mastrangelo, M., & Turnbull, D. (2021). The impact of surgically diagnosed symptomatic endometriosis on women's social lives, work and education: An inductive classical content analysis. *Australian and New Zealand Journal of Obstetrics and Gynecology.* https://doi.org/10.1111/ajo.13447

McCool, M. E., Zuelke, A., Theurich, M. A., Knuettel, H., Ricci, C., & Apfelbacher, C. (2016). Prevalence of female sexual dysfunction among premenopausal women: A systematic review and meta-analysis of observational studies. *Sexual Medicine Reviews, 4*(3), 197–212.

McDonald, E. A., Gartland, D., Small, R., & Brown, S. J. (2016). Frequency, severity and persistence of postnatal dyspareunia to 18 months post partum: A cohort study. *Midwifery, 34,* 15–20. doi:10.1016/j. midw.2016.01.012

Meana, M. (2012). *Sexual dysfunction in women.* Hogrefe Publishing.

Moyal-Barracco, M., & Lynch, P. J. (2004). 2003 ISSVD terminology and classification of vulvo-dynia: A historical perspective. *Journal of Reproduction Medicine, 49,* 772–777.

Norinho, P., Martins, M. M., & Ferreira, H. (2020). A systematic review on the effects of endometriosis on sexuality and couple's relationship. *Facts, Views & Vision in Obstetrics and Gynaecology, 12*(3), 197–205.

Parasar, P., Ozcan, P., & Terry, K. L. (2017). Endometriosis: Epidemiology, diagnosis and clinical management. *Current Obstetrics and Gynecology Reports, 6*(1), 34–41. doi:10.1007/s13669-017-0187-1

Paulson, J. D., & Delgado, M. (2007). The relationship between interstitial cystitis and endometriosis in patients with chronic pelvic pain. *JSLS: Journal of the Society of Laparoendoscopic Surgeons, 11*(2), 175–181.

Pelvic Floor First. (2019, January 15). *The hypertonic pelvic floor.* Retrieved December 23, 2020, from www.pelvicfloorfirst.org.au/news/577/ the-hypertonic-pelvic-floor

Poll, M. V., Barneveld, E. V., Aerts, L., Maas, J. W., Lim, A. C., Greef, B. T., . . . Hanegem, N. V. (2020). Endometriosis and sexual quality of life. *Sexual Medicine, 8*(3), 532–544. doi:10.1016/j.esxm.2020.06.004

Pukall, C. F., Goldstein, A. T., Bergeron, S., Foster, D., Stein, A., Kellogg-Spadt, S., . . . Bachmann, G. (2016a). Vulvodynia: Definition, prevalence, impact and pathophysiological factors. *Journal of Sexual Medicine, 13*(3), 291–304.

Raizada, V., & Mittal, R. K. (2008). Pelvic floor anatomy and applied physiology. *Gastroenterology Clinics of North America, 37*(3), 493–509. doi:10.1016/j.gtc.2008.06.003

Reed, D., Harlow, S. D., Sen, A., Legocki, L. J., Edwards, R. M., Arato, N., & Haefner, H. K. (2012). Prevalence and demographic characteristics of vulvodynia in a population-based sample. *American Journal of Obstetrics and Gynecology, 206*(2). doi:10.1016/j.ajog.2011.08.012

Reissing, E., Binik, Y., Khalifé, S., Cohen, D., & Amsel, R. (2004). Vaginal spasm, pain, and behavior: An empirical investigation of the diagnosis of vaginismus. *Archives of Sexual Behavior, 33,* 5–17. doi:10.1023/ B:ASEB.0000007458.32852.c8

Reissing, E., Borg, C., Spoelstra, S., ter Kuile, M., Both, S., De Jong, P., . . . Weijmar Schultz, W. (2014). "Throwing the baby out with the bathwater": The demise of vaginismus in favor of Genito-pelvic pain/ penetration disorder. *Archives of Sexual Behavior, 43*, 1209–1213. doi:10.1007/s10508-014-0322-2

Ribeiro, H. S., Paiva, A. M., Taliberti, B. da, Gonçalves, A. L., Condes, R. P., & Ribeiro, P. A. (2021). Psychological problems experienced by patients with bowel endometriosis awaiting surgery. *Revista Brasileira De Ginecologia e Obstetrícia/RBGO Gynecology and Obstetrics, 43*(09), 676–681. https://doi.org/10.1055/s-0041-1735938

Schneider, M. P., Vitonis, A. F., Fadayomi, A. B., Charlton, B. M., Missmer, S. A., & Divasta, A. D. (2020). Quality of life in adolescent and young adult women with dyspareunia and endometriosis. *Journal of Adolescent Health, 67*(4), 557–561. doi:10.1016/j.jadohealth.2020.02.024

Signorello, L. B., Harlow, B. L., Chekos, A. K., & Repke, J. T. (2001). Postpartum sexual functioning and its relationship to perineal trauma: A retrospective cohort study of primiparous women. *Transactions of the Nineteenth Annual Meeting of the American Gynecological and Obstretrical Society, 184*(5), 881–890. doi:10.1067/mob.2001.113855

Soliman, A. M., Rahal, Y., Robert, C., Defoy, I., Nisbet, P., Leyland, N., & Singh, S. (2021). Impact of ENDOMETRIOSIS On fatigue and Productivity impairment in a cross-sectional survey of Canadian women. *Journal of Obstetrics and Gynaecology Canada, 43*(1), 10–18. doi:10.1016/j. jogc.2020.06.022

Soliman, A. M., Surrey, E., Bonafede, M., Nelson, J. K., & Castelli-Haley, J. (2018). Real-world evaluation of direct and indirect economic burden among endometriosis patients in the United States. *Advances in Therapy, 35*(3), 408–423. doi:10.1007/s12325-018-0667-3

Sparks, H. (2020, November 10). *Millions of women don't know where their own vagina is located.* Retrieved December 28, 2020, from https://nypost.com/2020/11/10/millions-of-women-dont-know-where-their-own-vagina-is-located/

ter Kuile, M., Bulté, I., Weijenborg, P., Beekman, A., Melles, R., & Onghena, P. (2009). Therapist-aided exposure for women with lifelong vaginismus: A replicated single-case design. *Journal of Consulting and Clinical Psychology, 77*, 149–159. doi:10.1037/a0014273 ter Kuile, M., & Reissing, E. (2014). Lifelong vaginismus. In Y. Binik & K. Hall (Eds.), *Principles and practice of sex therapy* (5th ed.). The Guilford Press.

ter Kuile, M. M., Melles, R. J., Tuijnman, R. C. C., de Groot, H. E., & van Lankveld, J. J. D. M. (2015). Therapist aided exposure for women with lifelong vaginismus: Mediators of treatment outcome: A randomized waiting list control trial. *Journal of Sexual Medicine, 12*(8), 1807–1819. doi:10.1111/jsm.12935

van der Velde, J., Laan, E., & Everaerd, W. (2001). Vaginismus, a component of a general defensive reaction: An investigation of pelvic floor muscle activity during exposure to emotion-inducing film excerpts in women with and without vaginismus. *International Urogynecology Journal and Pelvic Floor Dysfunction, 12*, 328–331.

van Lankveld, J. J., Brewaeys, A. M., ter Kuile, M., & Weijenborg, P. (1995). Difficulties in the differential diagnosis of vaginismus, dyspareunia and mixed sexual pain disorder. *Journal of Psychosomatic Obstetrics & Gynecology, 16*, 201–209. doi:10.3109/01674829509024470

van Lankveld, J. J., Granot, M., Weijmar Schultz, W. C., Binik, Y. M., Wessleman, U., Pukall, C. F., & Achtrari, C. (2010). Women's sexual pain disorders. *Journal of Sexual Medicine, 7*, 615–631.

Vlaeyen, J., & Linton, S. (2000). Fear-avoidance and its consequences in chronic musculoskeletal pain: A state of the art. *Pain, 85*, 317–332. doi:10.1016/S0304-3959(99)00242-0

Witzeman, K., Flores, O. A., Renzelli-Cain, R. I., Worly, B., Moulder, J. K., Carrillo, J. F., & Schneider, B. (2020). Patient – physician interactions regarding dyspareunia with endometriosis: Online survey results. *Journal of Pain Research, 13*, 1579–1589. doi:10.2147/jpr.s248887

Wu, J. M., Vaughan, C. P., Goode, P. S., Redden, D. T., Burgio, K. L., Richter, H. E., & Markland, A. D. (2014). Prevalence and trends of symptomatic pelvic floor disorders in U.S. Women. *Obstetrics & Gynecology, 123*(1), 141–148. doi:10.1097/aog.0000000000000057

Zimmermann, A., Bernuit, D., Gerlinger, C., Schaefers, M., & Geppert, K. (2012). Prevalence, symptoms and management of uterine fibroids: An international internet-based survey of 21,746 women. *BMC Women's Health, 12*(1). doi:10.1186/1472-6874-12-6

# 3

## UNWANTED SEXUAL EXPERIENCES AND SEXUAL VIOLENCE AGAINST WOMEN IN THE UNITED STATES

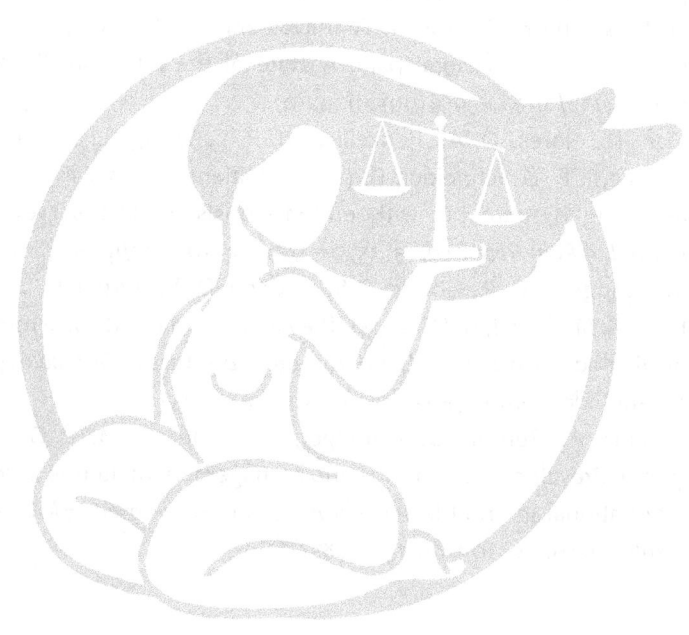

DOI: 10.4324/9781003168232-3

## Trends in the United States

Before we address the parallel experiences of seeking diagnosis and treatment for a pelvic/sexual pain disorder and sexual trauma, clinicians need to be aware of the prevalence of sexual violence against women in the United States. If you work with women in any clinical setting, it is imperative to understand how common these experiences are across the lifespan, as well as the impact of unwanted sexual experiences on women's physical health and mental health. Clinicians should also understand the nuances of how these traumatic incidents inform how women may view themselves as sexual beings and may shape how they understand themselves in different roles such as a mother, a sister, a coworker, etc.

Sexual victimization tends to happen in women's formative years with one in nine girls reporting sexual abuse by an adult before the age of 18 (Finkelhor et al., 2014). In addition, girls ages 16 to 19 are four times more likely to experience a rape or sexual assault compared with the general population, and girls and women aged 12 to 34 are at the greatest risk for experiencing rape or sexual assault (Greenfeld, 1997). Among women who reported having experienced sexual harassment or assault, 57% of them reported their first incident by age 17 (Kearl, 2018). Of female rape victims, 79.8% experienced their first rape before the age of 25 (Black et al., 2011). For women who attend college, one in four will experience a sexual assault while at school (Cantor et al., 2020). Based on these statistics, for girls and women in the United States, unwanted sexual experiences and sexual violence are the social norm. They are a part of what shapes the female experience in this country.

Most acts of sexual violence against women in the United States are completed by someone the woman knows, creating not only a traumatic event but also an interpersonal trauma and betrayal. Among women who have been raped, 51.1% of women reporting being raped by an intimate partner and 40.8% by an acquaintance (Black et al., 2011). Another 16.1% of women reported experiencing sexual coercion, or repeated requests and significant pressure to engage in unwanted sexual activities, usually by someone in a position of influence or authority (Smith et al., 2018). Many women who have coercive sexual experiences struggle with how to label or name what has happened to them. Coercive sexual experiences often look like an inordinate or extreme amount of pressure for sex, usually after a period of "grooming," which makes the victim more vulnerable. The perpetrator is someone who has power of the victim such as a teacher, a coach, a boss or supervisor, an older peer, etc. They usually make the victim feel as though they are obligated to engage in sexual activity with them. The perpetrator may promise some kind of special treatment in return for sex such as a promotion, while others use threats of spreading lies or rumors about the victim to bully them into compliance.

The overwhelming majority of women in the United States are also subject to street harassment, often which escalates to the level of a sexual assault. The National Study on Sexual Harassment and Assault (2018) found that 81% of women experienced sexual harassment or sexual assault. Among women who experienced sexual harassment, 51% reported being touched without their consent, 34% were physically followed, and 30% of women experienced being flashed by the perpetrator. In terms of location of sexual harassment, 66% of women reported being sexually harassed in public spaces, 38% of women reported being sexually harassed at work, and 35% of women reported being sexually harassed at their residences (Kearl, 2018). In general, women of color are more likely than white women to experience a sexual assault, with Native American women being at the greatest risk (Department of Justice, 2004). Furthermore, bisexual women are at the greatest risk of sexual assault, followed by lesbian women and heterosexual women respectively.

## Context Matters: Understanding Institutional Betrayal

All these unwanted sexual experiences occur within a larger social context and within institutions such as higher education, medical systems, places of employment, religious institutions, etc. It is important to understand the role of these institutions in enabling or exacerbating trauma. I find the framework of institutional betrayal and other betrayal trauma theory extremely helpful in understanding the impact institutions can have on traumatic experiences. Smith and Freyd (1996, 2013) coined the term "institutional betrayal," which refers to "wrongdoings perpetrated by an institution upon individuals dependent on that institution, including failure to prevent or respond supportively to wrongdoings by individuals (e.g. sexual assault) committed within the context of the institution."

As discussed in Chapter 1, the Larry Nassar case is an example of institutional betrayal. Multiple organizations, from USA Gymnastics to the FBI to the University of Michigan, failed to intervene in stopping child sexual abuse despite their knowledge of its occurrence, allowing for hundreds of young women to be sexually abused over three decades. Another example of institutional betrayal is universities' complete failures to investigate reports of sexual assaults despite regulations of Title IX, with many survivors feeling blamed, penalized, and pushed out of their universities (Longman, 2022). Further complicating the barriers that many college students face when reporting sexual assaults are laws that treat survivors differently based on whether the survivor chose to consume alcohol or was forced to. In fact, 27 states still distinguish between survivors who chose to drink or use drugs and those who were forced to. These laws have implications for whether charges are even filed after a sexual assault has been reported. In many cases when women admit to having chosen to consume alcohol or drugs, no charges against the perpetrator will be filed (Elbeshbishi, 2022).

Part of institutional betrayal may involve "Institutional DARVO," which stands for "Deny, Attack, and Reverse Victim and Offender" (Freyd, 1997). DARVO happens on an individual level, like, for instance, when an abusive husband makes false allegations of abuse against his wife whom he is actually abusing. Institutional DARVO could look like a university penalizing a student for underage drinking after she reports a sexual assault. Women are more likely to experience DARVO than men during confrontations, and it contributes to self-blame among victims (Harsey et al., 2017). DARVO often feels like gaslighting and leaves those on the receiving end disoriented and fearful, especially when it involves manipulation of the legal system. For instance, when Noemi reported her sexual assault to her company's human resources department, the company engaged in institutional DARVO. They denied the event occurred, basing their conclusion on Mr. X's recollection of events only, and then questioned her motives to bring harm Mr. X's reputation, questioned whether she had sexual relationships with others in the company, etc.

Research has demonstrated the broad negative impact of institutional betrayal. Institutional betrayal has been linked to higher levels of post-traumatic symptoms in sexual assault survivors and sexual dysfunction (Smith & Freyd, 2013). A study of college students who had experienced trauma found that institutional betrayal was associated with a range of health problems and dissociative symptoms (Smith & Freyd, 2017). Institutional betrayal may also impact victims' educational attainment, career paths, and financial stability if consequences of the institutional betrayal cause them to leave or change schools and careers. In Noemi's case, she was forced out of a promising position at a large company and believed this had long-term negative consequences on her career.

Given the negative impacts on mental health, physical health, and quality of life, it is important to assess for betrayal trauma with any client seeking treatment for a traumatic event. Clinicians should assess for the many layers of betrayal, which include institutional betrayal, family betrayal, betrayal by peers, societal or cultural betrayal, and spiritual betrayal (for more in-depth information, refer to Chapter 4). For each type of betrayal, you want to assess the "ripple effects" – or the series of related consequences caused by the betrayal. Without family or peer support, for instance, some women may experience depression or anxiety due to their family members or peers not believing their disclosure. Unfortunately, I have also seen some cases when a family may decide to withdraw financial support for a college or graduate student if the woman has disclosed sexual abuse within the family. An example that many of my clients have experienced as societal or cultural betrayal was the media spectacle and reactions around the Brett Kavanaugh case. Many clients cited this case in particular as why they would not report their unwanted sexual experiences. In their view, the perpetrator received his promotion. Meanwhile the victim received death threats, was character assassinated, had to relocate herself and her family, and was unable to return to her job because of speaking about her unwanted sexual experience.

For religious clients, a traumatic event can cause a spiritual crisis and a sense of feeling betrayed by their higher power, causing some survivors to question their entire belief system. For survivors whose unwanted sexual experiences have occurred by a spiritual leader or someone affiliated with their religious organization, the betrayal can feel even more disorienting. It is also important to note both actual betrayal as well as anticipated betrayal have similar consequences. Many college students never disclose their sexual assaults on campus because they anticipate not being believed by their administrations. The anticipation of not being believed or supported usually comes from real events the client has witnessed or experienced. For instance, Violet had heard of other students reporting sexual assaults but also knew the perpetrators remained on campus, while most of the rumored victims seemed to leave. For someone like Violet relying on scholarship to fund her education, she worried about the consequences of reporting.

In Paula's case, she experienced institutional betrayal from both her school and the legal system. Her school initially failed to protect her from a predatory teacher and coach. Perhaps it could be argued that the school could not have known the teacher was pursuing a sexual and romantic relationship with a teenage student (despite some very obvious red flags). Fine. However, their response once criminal charges were filed against the teacher after an extensive investigation was to initially defend and protect the teacher. While this teacher sat at home continuing to collect a salary for another year, the school also failed to address the cyber bullying of Paula by her peers. Eventually, the school fired the predatory teacher but for a much lesser charge and not for anything related to the sexual abuse. In fact, the school refused to acknowledge the abuse even once the teacher was found criminally guilty and sentenced by the state.

A mandated reporter made the initial report to the state's child abuse reporting hotline. While the criminal investigation was triggering, what was more upsetting for Paula was having her personal character attacked by the defense attorney and feeling pressured by almost everyone involved in the case to advocate for less severe charges for her perpetrator because she "wanted the relationship at one point." This harmful stance not only ignored the powerful impact of grooming, but it also ignored the role of obvious and inappropriate power dynamics (teacher–student, and significant age differences). Paula never regretted her disclosure per se to the mandated reporter, which led to the criminal case against her teacher, but she did feel failed by the legal system. Despite the clear and significant evidence, the case dragged on for years. Family members of the perpetrators harassed her online, and one even showed up on her college campus looking for her. Another family member of the perpetrator showed up at her family's house, making threats to her parents. Others in her community accused her "seeking revenge" and "just wanting money." The character attacks baffled Paula given that it was not her decision to report and that the criminal case did not involve any financial compensation for her. Paula eventually stopped going home due to the hostile environment, and her parents quickly sold their home of over 20 years to relocate out of state.

## Important Considerations in Working With Sexual Trauma Survivors in the #MeToo Era

It is important for clinicians to be familiar with the unique concerns that many survivors today face:

1. *The resurfacing of similar betrayals:* As previously discussed, survivors are likely to have multiple layers of betrayal related to the trauma. These betrayals may also parallel other struggles they have had in their lives, creating more distress for the client. Violet feared being dismissed by the administration at her university if she reported the sexual assault. Unfortunately, Violet's existence as a child was also dismissed by her biological father's family because she was the product of an affair. She also felt her black identity was ignored by the white family that raised her. So, when she was later dismissed by healthcare providers about her severe pelvic pain and period pain, she was already used to being treated this way, contributing to feeling helpless. The treatment by the healthcare providers did stir up the old wounds from childhood regarding both sides of her family's treatment of her. To understand these parallel experiences, clinicians should always conduct a thorough history with the client, as this will often inform the clinician about the lens from which the client will experience their trauma. The next chapter discusses in detail the "parallel pain" of unwanted sexual experiences and the process of getting diagnosed and treated for a pelvic/ sexual pain disorder.

2. *Expressing anger:* I often see women mislabel any feelings of anger as being "out of control" or "bad." Even when women can recognize their anger as valid, it may still feel scary and unacceptable. What

I think these survivors are reacting to is the lifelong message that women are not allowed to be angry, and if they are angry, they're "crazy" or "mean." Some of this mislabeling is due to the real social penalty for women who express anger. If anger is suppressed, it may turn into depression or anxiety or sit somewhere physically in the body like, for instance, the pelvis. Therefore, part of our role as clinicians is helping women to access and express their anger appropriately and healthily. Sometimes even appropriate and healthy expressions of anger still result in a social penalty, like, for instance, being accused of being abusive, a common reaction from narcissistic men when faced with women's valid anger. Clinicians should be able to provide psychoeducation about the social penalty of anger and help clients way the options for assertively expressing anger. At her perpetrator's sentencing, Paula decided to share her victim's statement as she believed it important to her healing. In this statement, she expressed her anger, as Paula had many valid reasons to be angry. She was assertive during her statement, raising her voice occasionally, but did not curse or act out in an inappropriate way. Despite this, a few of the local newspapers reporting on the story described her presentation as "bitter" and "unhinged." This experience was retraumatizing for Paula, who felt judged and blamed throughout the entire ordeal.

3. *Reconciling "good girl" behavior:* Clinicians may need to help survivors address "good girl" behavior that may have put them at risk for experiencing unwanted sexual experiences. Women are still socialized to be accommodating to others and to put other's needs before their own. As a child, this might look like being told to give a relative a hug or kiss despite not wanting to or playing the games siblings or friends wish to play instead of what you would like to do. A childhood of these seemingly small acts sets women up for poor boundary setting and difficulties with being assertive as a teen and adult. In dating, these behaviors could put a woman more at risk for coercive sexual experiences or sexual assault. It also may look like putting up with behaviors in romantic relationships that are not okay, whether being the default parent or person who does all of the household management or being taken advantage of financially or sexually. Sometimes survivors recollect knowing something was

off about the perpetrator but ignored their gut feelings because they did not want to make the perpetrator "feel bad." Others feel pressured to play along with sexual advances or simply comply. This can be disorienting, angering, and painful when women start to connect how gender socialization by family and culture may have set them up for unwanted sexual experiences or abuse. Women may need to decide if they want to modify certain behaviors, like, for instance, learning to be more assertive sexually and in general.

4. *Allowing space for grief:* Once survivors' posttraumatic stress disorder (PTSD)–like symptoms have subsided and they are no longer in crisis, grief of "what could have been" is likely to set in. Helping survivors process this grief is imperative for healing and for envisioning a future (something those with PTSD can often struggle with). The more layers of betrayal, the more grief I typically see, as the ripple effects of the trauma has impacted many areas of the person's life. After Rebecca had processed her traumatic memories from childhood about being abused by her older brother and her recent accident and medical trauma, she felt overwhelmed by grief. She had to grieve for the child who never knew safety in her home and the cascading consequences, realizing that she never truly had been able to be a child or teenager.

5. *Toxic positivity around forgiveness:* I have often heard survivors distressed about their inability to "forgive" as if it is necessary condition to heal. Violet felt pressure to "forgive and move on" after she did disclose her sexual assault to a few peers. The burden of "needing to forgive in order to heal" made her feel, "like it was my fault that I was still bothered by what had happened. Almost as if I were giving permission to a ghost to haunt me." Women survivors particularly, more so than men survivors, I believe, experience social and cultural pressure to forgive. While forgiveness may be a part of some survivors' healing journeys, it is not a part of everyone's journey. Survivors should not be misled to believe they must forgive in order to heal. Survivors should also understand that the act of forgiving may not necessarily lead to the expectations they have around forgiveness (which can be unrealistic). This toxic positivity message can create more distress for women who already experience self-blame.

6.   *Support and explore all options:* I believe our role as clinicians is to support and explore all options with clients, even ones we ourselves would never entertain. It is ultimately the survivor's choice who they want to disclose their story to and how they want to tell their story. Realizing that they now have control over the narrative of their unwanted sexual experience and can decide who will know about this experience can be empowering for survivors. It is often helpful to explain that disclosure of their experiences can happen on a spectrum and that they can approach disclosure on a case-by-case basis. The reality is that survivors may have many people in their lives who, at best, might not be supportive and, at worst, openly hostile towards the survivor, especially if the perpetrator is in the family or a close friend. There are real consequences to disclosing sexual abuse or assault, especially in a society that blames women and provides little support for survivors. I have had clients whose families cut them off after reporting sexual abuse. Others, like Noemi, have lost jobs or roles that were extremely important to them. Sadly, I have even seen a few cases when a former spouse will cite the sexual abuse or sexual assault as justification for custody. Given the dismal outcomes in our justice system for survivors, therapists also need to communicate that it is a survivor's choice whether they want to pursue legal action or not against the perpetrator (with the exception, of course, being those whose abuse was reported by a mandated reporter). It is the client's choice whether they want to subject themselves to our current legal system or not, and having a case tried legally is not necessary to feeling validated or to heal from the trauma.

7.   *Providing support through continued betrayal:* Survivors may report their unwanted sexual experiences to authority figures but in most cases will endure additional trauma as a result. Survivors whose cases end up in the criminal justice system should be prepared for the likely vicious attacks by the defense and media. Clinicians who are working with survivors whose cases are possibly going to trial need to be extra diligent about documentation in case they are subpoenaed. Paula's case highlighted the continued betrayal and trauma many survivors face during legal proceedings and media attention. Paula described the treatment by the justice system and media as

upsetting and traumatizing as the sexual abuse she endured. Given this, she needed additional support and therapeutic interventions that addressed these painful ripple effects from the original trauma.

8.  *Preparing clients for publicity or media impact:* For survivors whose cases or stories have been made public, whether by their own choice or not, social media and online commentary on articles featuring their experiences can be particularly brutal. While victims of sexual abuse are often anonymous in the media, the pain of knowing how negatively you're being portrayed by the media can be highly distressing. I have yet to work with a client who felt they had been fairly painted in the media. Most experience the coverage at best as distorted and, at worst, a vicious character assassination. It is helpful to warn clients about how they may feel reading about themselves and their stories in the media. The pros and cons of exposing oneself to these stories should also be weighed with the client.

## The Therapist as the Witness, Ally, and Survivor

Given how common unwanted sexual experiences are for women, it is likely that you may have had unwanted sexual experiences or have close friends or family members who have had unwanted sexual experiences. As a therapist and fellow human, we play the role of witness – to others unwanted sexual experiences – by listening to their stories or being a bystander to these events. We may also play the role of the ally – as someone who perhaps is involved in helping those to heal from unwanted sexual experiences and advocating for survivors in both our personal and professional lives. And finally, we may also play the role of survivor – which may make us understand the experiences of our clients more deeply but make us more vulnerable to feeling triggered by our clients' stories.

These multiple roles in multiple settings can be difficult to balance at times. Signs that you may be struggling with this balance include ruminating about a particular case, experiencing symptoms of burnout, feeling hypervigilant or on edge, having nightmares about the details of a case, or having intense emotional reactions about a case that are impacting your own ability to manage your emotions during session with a client. If you are a trauma survivor, it is normal to feel triggered by hearing a client's story. However, if these triggers persist and begin to negatively impact your ability to be present for clients or are making life outside of work more difficult to manage, then intervention for yourself is likely needed. As clinicians, it is imperative that we monitor for, and try to prevent, burnout. We need to make sure our own mental health is in a stable place to help others heal.

To prevent burnout around trauma-related cases, I recommend capping the number of capital "T" trauma-related cases (rape, sexual assault, combat trauma, other violent assaults) on your caseload at one time. Given the potential for significant additional work, I also recommend clinicians take no more than one or two trauma cases in which the legal system is involved. While clients certainly change their minds through the process of therapy and may decide to either pursue to drop their legal cases, capping legal related cases at one to two clients at a time will help you to manage this burden to some degree. Finally, if you work with capital "T" trauma cases, I recommend seeking regular supervision for these cases.

When juggling these multiple roles of the witness, ally, and survivor, you may find you need to step back or remove yourself from a role to prevent burnout. For instance, it is common for clinicians who work with capital "T" trauma sexual assault cases to need boundaries outside of work regarding this topic. Sometimes this may just mean avoiding TV shows or movies in which this is the featured theme. Other times clinicians may find themselves needing a break from the role of "ally" outside of work. So, while your non-clinician allies may have the energy to go to a march against rape and sexual assault or help to edit a memo advocating for more effective political policies for sexual assault and rape survivors, it is okay if you do not.

Sometimes despite our best efforts to prevent burnout or distress related to trauma cases, we may find ourselves exactly in that position. A clinician working with significant trauma cases may find it useful to seek therapy themselves because secondary trauma can occur because of treating clients who have experienced trauma. I highly recommend eye movement desensitization and reprocessing for clinicians experiencing symptoms of secondary trauma. If you find yourself overwhelmed, put a pause on accepting new clients. And finally, it is always okay and sometimes the most ethical action to take to refer a client to another clinician if you find yourself too burned out or triggered by a particular case. It is also okay to take a more extended break from capital "T" trauma cases. Treating survivors is extremely important work; however, it must be done at a sustainable pace. Each clinician must find the pace that is most manageable for them given the other roles and stressors they are balancing in their own lives.

## Important Takeaways

- Unwanted sexual experiences are extremely common for girls and women in the United States. Many women have experienced multiple instances of sexual trauma over their lifespan.
- Sexual trauma always occurs within a larger social context, and survivors may experience betrayal traumas on many levels.
- Survivors who experience institutional betrayal are at greater risk for negative impacts to physical health, mental health, and financial stability.
- Clinicians may be juggling roles of being a survivor themselves, being a witness, and being an ally. Balancing these roles can sometimes be challenging, and clinicians need to be mindful of self-care, knowing their own limitations and signs of burnout.

## References

Black, M. C., Basile, K. C., Breiding, M. J., Smith, S. G., Walters, M. L., Merrick, M. T., Chen, J., & Stevens, M. R. (2011). *The national intimate partner and sexual violence survey (NISVS): 2010 summary report.* National Center for Injury Prevention and Control, Centers for Disease Control and Prevention. www.cdc.gov/violenceprevention/pdf/NISVS_Report2010-a.pdf

Cantor, D., Fisher, B., Chibnall, S., Harps, S., Townsend, R., Thomas, G., . . . Madden, K. (Revised January 17, 2020). *Report on the AAU campus climate survey on sexual assault and misconduct.* Prepared by Westat for The Association of American Universities.

Department of Justice. (2004). *Office of justice programs, Bureau of justice statistics.* American Indians and Crime, 1992–2002.

Elbeshbishi, S. (2022, January 18). How sexual assault victims became incapacitated often decides charges. *USA Today.* Retrieved January 22,

2022, from www.usatoday.com/web-stories/how-sexual-assault-victims-became-incapacitated-often-decides-charges/

Finkelhor, D., Shattuck, A., Turner, H. A., & Hamby, S. L. (2014). The lifetime prevalence of child sexual abuse and sexual Assault assessed in late adolescence. *Journal of Adolescent Health*, 55(3), 329–333. doi:10.1016/j.jadohealth.2013.12.026

Freyd, J. J. (1996). *Betrayal trauma: The logic of forgetting childhood abuse.* Harvard University Press.

Freyd, J. J. (1997). Ii. violations of power, adaptive blindness and betrayal trauma theory. *Feminism & Psychology*, 7(1), 22–32. doi:10.1177/0959353597071004

Freyd, J. J. (2008, March 6). *The psychology of betrayal trauma: Memory, health, and gender.* Lecture, Thompson Hall Science and Mathematics Seminar, University of Puget Sound.

Freyd, J. J. (2008, April 11). *Betrayal trauma: Memory, health, and gender.* Colloquium, Department of Psychology, New Mexico State University.

Greenfeld, L. A. (1997). *Sex offenses and offenders: An analysis of data on rape and sexual assault.* Department of Justice, Office of Justice Programs, Bureau of Justice Statistics.

Harsey, S. J., Zurbriggen, E. L., & Freyd, J. J. (2017). Perpetrator responses to victim confrontation: Darvo and victim self-blame. *Journal of Aggression, Maltreatment & Trauma*, 26(6), 644–663. doi:10.1080/10926771.2017.1320777

Kearl, H. (2018, February). *Stop street harassment. The facts behind the #MeToo movement: A national study on sexual harassment and assault.* https://stopstreetharassment.org/wp-content/uploads/2018/01/Full-Report-2018-National-Study-on-Sexual-Harassment-and-Assault.pdf

Longman, M. (2022, January 5). *She reported her rape to her college. what happened next left her devastated.* How Does Title IX Work on College Campuses Now? Report. Retrieved January 22, 2022, from www.refinery29.com/en-us/2022/01/10666176/title-ix-9-college-campus-sexual-assault-cases

Smith, C. P., & Freyd, J. J. (2013). Dangerous safe havens: Institutional betrayal exacerbates sexual trauma. *Journal of Traumatic Stress*, 26(1), 119–124. doi:10.1002/jts.21778

Smith, C. P., & Freyd, J. J. (2014). Institutional betrayal. *American Psychologist*, 69(6), 575–587. doi:10.1037/a0037564

Smith, C. P., & Freyd, J. J. (2017). Insult, then injury: Interpersonal and institutional betrayal linked to health and dissociation. *Journal of Aggression, Maltreatment & Trauma, 26*(10), 1117–1131. doi:10.1080/10 926771.2017.1322654

Smith, S. G., Zhang, X., Basile, K. C., Merrick, M. T., Wang, J., Kresnow, M., & Chen, J. (2018). *The national intimate partner and sexual violence survey (NISVS): 2015 data brief – updated release.* National Center for Injury Prevention and Control, Centers for Disease Control and Prevention. www.cdc.gov/violenceprevention/pdf/2015data-brief508.pdf

Walters, M. L., Chen, J., & Breiding, M. J. (2013). *The national intimate partner and sexual violence survey (NISVS): 2010 findings on victimization by sexual orientation.* National Center for Injury Prevention and Control Centers for Disease Control and Prevention Atlanta.

# 4

## PARALLEL PAIN

### Pelvic/Sexual Pain and Unwanted Sexual Experiences

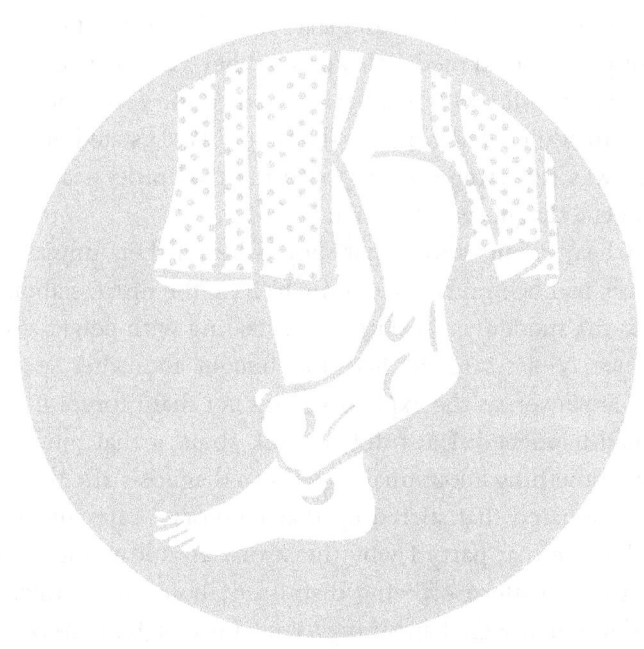

DOI: 10.4324/9781003168232-4

## The Same Pain

Women's experiences with sexual trauma often parallel their process of trying to obtain a diagnosis or seek treatment for a pelvic/sexual pain disorder. It is because of these parallels that the two experiences can trigger and exacerbate each other. Paula sought the opinion of her OB/GYN about the pain she was having when attempting to have sex with her boyfriend. The doctor initially reassured her that the pain was "normal if you're new to sex." Paula explained that the pain didn't seem to be like the "normal pain" her friends talked about when they had sex for the first time and that she was worried something else was wrong. The doctor then snapped back, "Well, maybe you don't know what you're doing when it comes to having sex." Paula left without answers for her pelvic/sexual pain and felt blamed for her symptoms.

Paula was also preparing for the criminal trial against her former teacher/coach. Just like at the OB/GYN office, the process made her feel like she was to blame. Peers from her high school sent her "really, really, really mean DMs" about how she must have "wanted it" and "snitched" after the teacher broke up with her. Despite the obvious power differentials, a 15-year age difference and state laws that forbid teacher–student relationships, the local media also painted her as a scorned lover out for revenge – not a child who had been groomed for years and then sexual abused by an adult. "The blame is the same," Paula stated during session when she was reflecting on how both the trial process and process of trying to get a diagnosis felt similar.

I often hear clients admit that they believed their unwanted sexual experiences had been processed, only to have the distress about the past sexual trauma suddenly resurface while dealing with pelvic/sexual pain. For instance, Violet said she had not thought about her sexual assault for years. However, as she explained, "It's not that I forgot it [the sexual assault] had happened; I just didn't think about it that much anymore. But it was something about finally getting a diagnosis after over a decade of being dismissed that stirred up that memory." Later in therapy, she came to believe that part of why the sexual assault memory resurfaced was due to the pattern of being dismissed about "real things that had happened to me or were happening to me. I was right. I knew something was wrong with me medically even though the doctors told me I was fine, and I knew the sexual assault had happened and was wrong even though the college administration ignored it."

Memories of past sexual assaults might also resurface due to the symptoms of physical pain in the pelvis. The body can store our memories and our traumas neurologically. When faced with similar sensations, the memories of past traumas may return. This can be scary and overwhelming for clients who believed they had already overcome the traumatic event. Rebecca's nervous system seemed to be stuck in a traumatic state after having a skiing accident that left her with chronic pelvic pain. Struggling with daily chronic pelvic pain felt eerily like her childhood in which she suffered chronic psychological, physical, and sexual abuse. Although she hadn't thought regularly about these memories since leaving her childhood home, she found herself thinking about them often since the onset of her pelvic pain. Although less common, for other clients with repressed memories of sexual violence, the symptoms of their pelvic/sexual pain disorder can sometimes bring these memories into focus.

As part of the research for my book, I conducted an online survey with women who had pelvic/sexual pain disorders. I was especially interested in understanding the similarities and differences between women with pelvic/sexual pain disorders who had unwanted sexual experiences and those who did not. Of the 175 survey participants, 56% reported having had an unwanted sexual experience. No difference between the two groups in the total number of pelvic/sexual pain diagnoses were found. However, women who endorsed having unwanted sexual experiences endured longer wait times for their diagnoses, had an earlier onset of pain, and saw more healthcare providers before receiving a diagnosis. In addition, of women who reported an unwanted sexual experience, 70% felt triggered by their sexual trauma during the diagnosis and treatment of their pelvic/sexual pain disorder.

There is little research regarding the possible implications of these findings. Based on my clinical experiences with women who have had both unwanted sexual experiences and have a pelvic/sexual pain disorder, many discuss the process of diagnosing and treating their condition as being very triggering. Feeling triggered by the process often results in avoiding or delaying certain treatments, which in turn seems to exacerbate the pelvic/sexual disorders and contribute to greater psychological distress. This avoidance leads to a larger ripple effect of the consequences from both the pelvic/sexual pain disorder and unwanted sexual experiences. It also leads to women feeling overwhelmed by ever growing barriers to treating both pelvic/sexual pain and trauma.

## Layers of Betrayal

In assessing women's current stressors who are seeking therapy for unwanted sexual experiences and/or pelvic/sexual pain I inventory the many "layers of betrayal" (Figure 4.1). Typically, the more layers of betrayal, the greater the distress. It is important to understand that betrayal can have actually occurred or was simply anticipated. For instance, as a child, Rebecca never disclosed the abuse she suffered at the hands of her older brother to her parents. She explained she anticipated either not being believed that the abuse was as bad as she was experiencing or that her parents would fail to take action to stop the abuse. As an adult, it was painful to realize her parents must have been aware of some level of abuse yet did little to protect her or her younger brother. Anticipated betrayal may have similar impacts to an actual betrayal, so it is important to assess and acknowledge anticipated betrayal. Violet experienced an actual betrayal when she reported the incident to her college and found herself questioned about binge drinking instead of addressing her assault.

The layers of betrayal include institutional betrayal, family betrayal, betrayal by peers, social/cultural betrayal, and spiritual betrayal. A more extensive discussion about institutional betrayal can be found in Chapter 3. In summary, institutional betrayal is the "wrongdoings perpetrated by an institution upon individuals dependent on that institution, including failure to prevent or respond supportively to wrongdoings by individuals (e.g. sexual assault) committed within the context of the institution" (Smith & Freyd, 2013). For example, Noemi faced institutional betrayal after disclosing her sexual assault, which happened at a work event by a superior. She was initially dismissed, then treated like as if she was the one who had done something wrong and pushed out of her job. After her postpartum hemorrhage, Noemi felt as though she "fell through the cracks" of the medical system during her aftercare,

# *Many layers of betrayal:*

*- Actual or anticipated*
*- More betrayal means more distress*

**Traumatic Event**

**Institutional**

**Family**

**Peers**

**Society/Culture**

**Spiritual**

especially after being ignored by doctors when she complained about having painful sex. The dismissals of her pelvic/sexual pain and resulting hopelessness felt very similar to the way her workplace treated her after disclosing the sexual assault.

Family betrayal could take many different forms, especially because sexual violence commonly occurs within the family. Sometimes families have patterns of inappropriate sexual behavior or sexual assaults over generations, especially if secret keeping and protection of the perpetrator have been modeled by previous generations. Often women who have been sexual violated within the family are not believed and face very high social penalties for confronting the abuse. One client I worked with explained that the risk of her disclosing the sexual abuse she suffered by her stepfather was quite high, as he was paying for her tuition. She anticipated her family not believing her and feared her family would stop paying for education, which jeopardized her ability to complete graduate school, as well as her long-term financial stability. Another client felt betrayed by her family after disclosing a sexual assault by her brother's friend. Although the sexual assault did not occur by a family member, the client was devastated that her family chose to believe her brother's friend's account of the event over her own. Women with pelvic/sexual pain disorders sometimes endure family betrayal in the form of lack of empathy or support. A client with severe endometriosis felt betrayed, and frankly abandoned, after her family refused to modify their adventurous vacations, resulting in her being unable to attend. Another woman with interstitial cystitis (IC) found herself teased by her in-laws regarding her frequent use of the bathroom. Sadly, her husband did not come to her defense but rather joined in on the jokes despite knowing the level of pain and embarrassment she was struggling with since having IC.

Peer betrayal can occur when friends, coworkers, neighbors, or other peers in a client's life fail to believe or support them. Paula encountered peer betrayal after classmates created a series of vicious social media accounts attacking her personally and her version of the sexual abuse. The lack of support at best, and at worst bullying, by the larger community eventually caused Paula's entire family to relocate out of state. Some women with pelvic/sexual pain disorders may come across a lack of support by peers. One client discussed the discomfort her friends expressed when she tried to share about the pain she had with sex after having her first baby. As she explained, "Since I was the first to have a baby in our friend group, maybe they didn't know how to relate, or maybe they were afraid that this could happen to them. Either way, their comments made me feel like damaged goods." Another client who needed an emergency hysterectomy after years of suffering from undiagnosed endometriosis felt extremely upset by her workplace's response. Despite needing a minimum six-week recovery, her boss expected her to be back in the office after two weeks and had sent an email to her coworkers implying that she was not in the office due to "emotional issues" – not due to a major surgery.

Social/cultural betrayal occurs from the larger social/cultural messages we receive. For instance, I have had many women survivors feel extremely triggered by the dynamics displayed at the Brett Kavanaugh hearing. This event represented their own experiences as survivors of sexual violence – that even if you're calm, well-spoken, and have collaborative evidence, you're likely to be the one who is punished. Ultimately, Brett Kavanaugh received his promotion despite lashing out at the hearing, and Dr. Christine Blasey Ford received death threats against her and her family and has not been able to return to work. Our culture continues to send victim-blaming messages about women who have faced sexual violence. Another example of social/cultural betrayal are the 27 state laws that mostly ignore women's reports of rape or sexual assault if they chose to consume alcohol or drugs (Elbeshbishi, 2022). For women with pelvic/sexual pain, social and cultural betrayal can look experiencing conflict in a romantic relationship due to sexual myths about women's sexual functioning that create unrealistic and unfair expectations.

Spiritual betrayal occurs when clients find themselves questioning their spiritual and religious beliefs after suffering a traumatic event. An unwanted sexual experience or struggling with a significant medical problem like pelvic/sexual pain can cause some to wonder how a higher power would allow such a thing to happen to them. Some question what they may have done to "deserve" such a difficulty or feel they have been cursed with bad luck. One devout client I worked with who developed pelvic/sexual pain after a medical trauma caused her to question her faith, which had previously been a large part of her identity. She also distanced herself from her religious community, which caused further isolation. Spiritual betrayal may be even more complex if the perpetrator is a religious leader or someone of power and importance in the client's faith-based community. The decision to report often feels very high stakes in these situations as clients risk jeopardizing losing their faith-based community and major source of social support.

## Betrayal Trauma in the Medical System

While there is a lack of research about comparing access and quality of care for women with different pelvic/sexual pain disorders, significant research does exist on the maternal mortality rate, which at least addresses the reproductive healthcare of women in the United States. The United States currently has the highest maternal mortality rate of any developed nation despite spending the highest percentage of its gross domestic product on healthcare. It is estimated that as many as two-thirds of the maternal deaths that occur in the United States are preventable (Melillo, 2020). While other developed nations have seen declining maternal mortality rates since the 1980s, the United States has seen their maternal mortality rate continue to increase (Kassebaum et al., 2016). The United States also has the lowest overall supply of midwives and OB/GYNs, with other developed nations having two to six times more than the United States. The United States is also the only high-income country that does not offer guaranteed paid leave for mothers (Melillo, 2020). Based on these indicators, pregnant and postpartum women in the United States are dealing with significant barriers to receiving adequate care.

Some existing research highlights the medical betrayal faced by women with pelvic/sexual pain disorders. In terms of pelvic/sexual pain disorders in women, it is extremely common for women to endure misdiagnosis. An online survey of 758 women with self-reported surgically confirmed endometriosis found an average diagnostic delay of 8.6 years, with 75.2% of women reporting being misdiagnosed with another physical health or mental health problem (Bontempo & Mikesell, 2020). These delays in appropriate diagnosis and treatment lead to negative long-term impacts on physical, emotional, relational, financial, professional, and sexual wellbeing. The consequences of these delays are often not able to be reversed, even once women receive an accurate diagnosis. In Violet's case, for instance, by the time she received a diagnosis for her endometriosis, the disease had already advanced to a severity that left her infertile and with daily chronic pain.

In tune with existing research, my online survey found an average diagnosis time of 5.4 years since first reporting symptoms, with participants seeing an average of 3.9 healthcare providers before receiving a diagnosis. In addition, there was a significant correlation between wait time and the impacts on romantic relationships, career, and financial stability. The longer the wait for a diagnosis, the greater the negative impact. What this means is the betrayal women encounter in the medical system effects more than their physical or emotional state but rather has long-term negative impacts on a women's quality of life.

## Barriers to Adequate Healthcare for Women With Pelvic/Sexual Pain Disorders

### *Cost of Treatment*

Sadly, for many women with pelvic/sexual pain disorders, the cost of treatment remains a significant barrier to treatment. Healthcare providers are left with few options for women when health insurance companies reimburse little in regard to pelvic/sexual pain. For instance, because Medicare views painful sex as a menopause-caused sexual dysfunction, it falls under the category of "lifestyle" conditions, and therefore related medical expenses are not covered (Kingsberg et al., 2019). Obviously, this decision also fails to acknowledge the large percentage of reproductive aged women struggling with pelvic/sexual pain conditions. The lack of insurance coverage forces women with pelvic/sexual pain disorders to take on a significant financial burden to treat their conditions. Only patients with extensive financial means will be able to afford the full range of necessary out-of-pocket expenses, including medications or injections and visits to pelvic/sexual pain specialists, pelvic floor physical therapists, and psychotherapists.

The cost of treatment and lack of insurance coverage also dictate the type of medical interventions that are available to women. However, the type of interventions women with pelvic/sexual pain receive have significant implications to the management of the condition and the quality of life. A study conducted in Spain that examined the long-term impact of laparoscopic excision of deep infiltrating endometriosis found that the sexual quality of life and health-related quality of life scores improved and were even similar to those of healthy women six months after surgery, with only a slight reduction of scores 36 months later (Martínez-Zamora et al., 2021). Unfortunately, in the United States, despite the evidence that excision surgery is more effective than ablation surgery, health insurance companies do not cover excision surgery. The lack of coverage stems from a 1992 Medicare Part B ruling that lumped all endometriosis surgery types together, including fulguration, ablation, coagulation, and excision. Health insurance companies determine how they will reimburse based on Medicare tables, which currently lack a code for excision surgery. Despite hundreds of clinical, peer-reviewed journals that demonstrate excision surgery's superiority over the other surgical options for endometriosis, the American Congress of Obstetricians and Gynecologists does not even recognize excision surgery as a specialty or the standard for treatment. Because of this, medical schools are not teaching excision surgery, resulting in few surgeons in the United States being able to perform such procedures (Cleary, 2018). This results in most women with endometriosis only being able to access subpar surgical interventions rather than what the research demonstrates works best.

Due to either poor insurance coverage or none at all for female pelvic/sexual pain conditions, many of my clients have to make very difficult decisions about what services or treatments to prioritize. The money they spend on out-of-pocket medical expenses related to their pelvic/sexual pain conditions has usually been diverted from other important expenses. Clients have told me the amount of money that they have had to spend on treating and managing their pelvic/sexual pain conditions has significantly impacted or prevented them from being able to save for retirement or retire, purchase a home, have children, return to school, and even pay for basic living expenses. The long-term financial stress related to managing and treating these conditions takes a negative toll emotionally and physically, only making these conditions more difficult to manage and exacerbating psychological distress.

As the wealth inequality continues to increase in the United States, I anticipate women will find it even more difficult to afford necessary medical treatment. I worry particularly for my clients younger than age

40, as both the Millennial Generation and Generation Z have significant financial barriers that previous generations have not faced, including being saddled with student debt and experiencing stagnant wages that have not kept up with the rapidly increasing cost of living, including the cost of childcare, healthcare, groceries, housing, etc. For example, since 1965, incomes have only increased by 15%, but home prices have increased 118% (Dickler, 2021). Traditionally, home ownership has served as a major financial asset for working and middle-class Americans but is now out of reach for most people younger than age 40. Research from Bain and Company on Generation Z and Millennial workers found that these employees face "slowing economic growth, rising inequality, and declining housing affordability." The report also found that "The odds of achieving absolute upward mobility – earning more than one's parents – are the lowest they have been in the US for any generation since World War II" (Jacob, 2022). These generations will age and with age will face health issues including pelvic/sexual pain. They will not, however, have the resources or assets that previous generations have been able to use to afford treatment.

My online survey found that 63% of respondents had significant difficulty or some difficulty with paying for out-of-pocket healthcare expenses related to their pelvic/sexual pain disorder. The average out-of-pocket expense spent on treatment was $4,900 and was significantly correlated with the number of healthcare providers seen. As already mentioned, my survey also found that the longer the wait time for a diagnosis, the greater the negative impact on the woman's career and financial stability. Pelvic/sexual pain disorders are extremely common, yet most women spend years being passed from specialist to specialist and, of course, spending money on these specialists. What my findings seem to highlight is that the common story of seeing multiple doctors over many years before receiving a diagnosis not only has a profound psychological impact but also has a significant impact negative on financial stability.

## The Burden of the Second Shift

Much of the burden of household management and childrearing, known as the "second shift," still falls on women. A United Nations report estimated that "women do 2.6 times the amount of unpaid and domestic work that men do." Another report by the US Department of Labor found that "men spend more time than women exercising, playing games and enjoying other leisure activities" (Carpenter, 2018). Girls and women are still socialized to put others' needs ahead of their own even when it negatively impacts their physical or emotional health. Because of the way women are socialized to be caregivers and men are also socialized to expect their female partners to be selfless, women are likely to take on more than they should in a relationship. A very common frustration I hear from my female clients in heterosexual relationships is that "all of the work" in the relationship falls on them – this often means the emotional work, household labor, childcare, logistics, scheduling, etc. This can lead women to feel burned out and resentful. It can also lead to poor physical and emotional health and low sexual desire.

Women in heterosexual relationships are often dealing with partners who engage in "weaponized incompetence," also known as "strategic incompetence." Whether consciously or unconsciously, this tactic is used by men to avoid household or childcare related tasks, contributing to the burden of the "second shift" for women. It often looks like men pretending they are unable to complete a task, or they attempt the task but do it so poorly or do not complete the job that the woman finds herself doing the task instead. For example, Siobhan vented in session that her husband "is an engineer who builds computers in his free time, yet somehow, can't start the laundry. He claims he's going to 'mess it up.' It's not that hard. Just look at the washing instructions on the tags! If I ask him to start dinner for us, he complains he doesn't know how, so he'll just order out for us. Then because I want to try and eat healthy, I end up cooking the meal anyway."

For women contending with a pelvic/sexual pain disorder, the impact of the second shift might specifically look like not being able to carve out the time to see a medical specialist or regularly attend pelvic floor physical therapy. Other women struggle with being able to create the time and privacy needed at home to engage in physical therapy exercises, dilators, or other exercises that help to improve or manage their pelvic/sexual pain conditions because they are taking on most of the childcare and household work. In addition, if women are burned out from the unequal distribution of labor at home, even if they have the time to engage in at home care, they often lack the energy.

Women with pelvic/sexual pain disorders might need to devote several hours a week to managing their condition in some way. But as their male partner, on the other hand, as Noemi explained, "All he has to do is show up with his erection." Without addressing the second shift and additional time needed to address the pelvic/sexual pain condition, resentment can quickly build. I have often seen cases in which the female partner finally reaches a place where she can physically have penetrative sex but feels so upset by the lack of support from her male partner throughout the process that she emotionally no longer wants to have sex with him.

### Physicians Without Knowledge of These Disorders

Most physicians receive little formal education and clinical experience in sexual health and sexual functioning. In fact, the time spent in medical school learning about sexual health and sexual functioning has decreased, and only a few residency programs include a focus on sexual medicine (Eardley et al., 2017; Shindel et al., 2016). A 2016 study using clinical case vignettes explored the comfort of 968 OB/GYN residents in taking a sexual history and providing counseling regarding the presenting concern. While two-thirds of the residents reported sexual health training being a priority in their residency, more than half of the residents were "unable to describe disorders of sexual function or list common medications that effect sexual function" (Worly et al., 2021). The lack of education and clinical experience later translates to an avoidance of discussing sexual health or sexual functioning with patients. Several studies have found that healthcare providers avoid addressing sexual health with their patients due to a lack of confidence regarding the topic, their own discomfort, perceiving discomfort from the patient, and lack of time during office visits (Kingsberg et al., 2019). Another study found that 73% of women reported that their primary care providers never asked about their sexual health or had only asked a few times (Fairchild et al., 2016).

Women in more rural settings may also lack access to specialists who can diagnosis and treat women with pelvic/sexual pain disorders.

Clinically, I have seen many women who did not receive a diagnosis until they ended up moving to a more urban area, where presumably there more specialists. Of note, my online survey did not find any differences between white women and BIPOC women in terms of wait time for a diagnosis or impact of the pelvic/sexual pain disorder on multiple life factors. However, women who identified as being from rural areas, versus suburban or urban areas, were found to have significantly longer wait times to receive a diagnosis. Further research would need to be done to explore this finding, but it perhaps is related to women in rural areas having less access to OB/GYNs who have knowledge of pelvic/ sexual pain disorders.

### Bias in the Healthcare System (Microaggressions!)

Microaggressions are intentional or unintentional negative messages that target a person based on their marginalized group status (such as race, gender, disability, sexual orientation, etc.). These messages can be verbal, nonverbal, or environmental (Sue & Spanierman, 2020). Many of the interactions with healthcare providers during the process of trying to find a diagnosis as described by my clients with pelvic/ sexual pain fit the definition of microaggressions. The general theme of these microaggressions seems to be related to the underlying biased and sexist beliefs that women are hysterical, do not know or understand their bodies, are weak, and have unrealistic expectations.

As part of my online survey, I asked respondent if they had been told by a healthcare provider during the process of getting a diagnosis or treatment for their pelvic/sexual pain disorder some of the most common microaggression examples I have heard from my clients. Of my survey respondents, 60.1% were told "I needed to relax," 51.7% that "The pain was normal," 42.1% that "The pain was in my head," and 39.9% that "There was no treatment for the pain." Another 30.9% of respondents had been told "I was overreacting," 21.4% "That having a child would cure or help my condition," and 19.1% "I had a low pain tolerance."

It should be of no surprise then, the findings from one study that found only 60% of women who reported chronic genital pain sought treatment, and 40% of these women never received a diagnosis (Harlow et al., 2001). Even when women do have the resources and courage to attempt to get their pelvic/sexual pain diagnosed, they find themselves at best dismissed and at worst bullied by their healthcare providers. It is in these microaggressions at the doctor's office that women who have experienced sexual trauma receive similar messaging about their experiences. The most common parallel messages about women's sexual trauma and pelvic/sexual pain I tend to hear are (1) You do not know your body/ are not the authority of your body, (2) You are not in power/control over body or life, (3) You are to blame for the trauma/medical issue, and (4) You are weak (you are suffering because you're not stronger). These messages create another layer of betrayal and psychological distress and interfere with women's ability to receive an accurate diagnosis and needed treatment. As already discussed, the delay in diagnosis greatly impacts women's long-term quality of life.

### Cumulative Effects of Misdiagnosis or Dismissal of Symptoms

It is common for women with pelvic/sexual pain to spend years in and out of doctors' offices seeking answers from specialists only to be misdiagnosed or dismissed. The cumulative impact of these experiences becomes a barrier. In the decade Violet spent searching for a diagnosis, she had been misdiagnosed on numerous occasions from everything from a sexually transmitted infection to somatization syndrome to chronic fatigue syndrome. Even though pain was Violet's most consistent and most intense symptom, she stated that the pain was rarely addressed. Through therapy, Violet and I explored the impact of doctors' attitudes towards her pain. She explained, "Because I was over and over denied help for my pain, I began to doubt my own pain. I took on their skepticism and tried to tell myself it wasn't real even though it felt real. Unfortunately, this allowed my endometriosis to grow."

Social stigma also dissuades many women from being able to bring up sexual concerns, including pelvic/sexual pain, with their healthcare providers. Several studies have confirmed that this avoidance and apprehension is consistent for women regardless of demographic factors such as race/ethnicity, age, education level, sexual orientation, and relationship status (Kingsberg et al., 2019). Many of the pelvic/sexual pain clients

I work with have the shared experience of finally pushing through the embarrassment and fear of being judged by a healthcare provider, only to have their concerns not addressed. After multiple incidents of being dismissed, many develop a "learned helplessness" mindset, preventing them from talking about their concerns.

By the time women with pelvic/sexual pain end up in my office, they often present with low self-esteem and difficulty trusting themselves partly due to the years of dismissals and misdiagnoses by healthcare providers. They often need to focus on basic assertiveness skill training to better communicate with their current treatment team. Commonly, clients also need help learning to trust their "gut" and own judgement again. If they stay in a learned helplessness mindset and are passive in their treatment, navigating treatment will prove extremely difficult even if they now have an effective treatment team.

## The Unfolding Impact of the COVID-19 Pandemic

The COVID-19 pandemic has created further delays in being able to receive a diagnosis or receive treatment. At both the onset of the pandemic and additional waves of increased infection, elective procedures have been canceled. Unfortunately, most surgeries and procedures related to diagnosing and treating pelvic/sexual pain are categorized as elective. The burden of the second shift has become even greater with children needing to attend virtual school from home, forcing many women to leave their jobs. Many of my pelvic/sexual pain clients had to pause their treatment due to being overwhelmed with household tasks and other COVID-related stressors. Others stopped treatment due to the fear of contracting the virus. Now two years into the pandemic as I write this chapter, many of them are now in poorer physical and mental health due to postponing treatment, on top of the additional stressors caused by the pandemic (lack of childcare, career demands or loss of job, lack of privacy and time for self-care, having fewer financial resources, etc.).

A recent study in Australia aimed to assess the impact of the pandemic on women with endometriosis. The study had 162 participants with an average age of 30.8 years old. Data were collected from participants at baseline and a 12-month follow-up. The study found that 60% of participants believed the pandemic negatively impacted their healthcare, with most participants experiencing a decline in their daily functioning. A logistic regression analysis was performed and found that the fear of COVID-19 also had a significant negative impact on participants' healthcare, symptoms, and daily functioning. Of importance, women living in areas that experienced the most serious lockdowns in Australia were significantly more impacted than women living in parts of Australia that did not have as extreme of lockdowns (Evans et al., 2021).

Clinicians must continue to assess for the impact of the pandemic on clients, especially for those with pelvic/sexual pain disorders. Generally, from my clients, there is a sense of dread and fear of what may happen next, especially given the pattern of some conditions improving with the pandemic only to then have the situation suddenly get worse again, like, for instance, when the delta and then omicron variants emerged. This psychological whiplash can make coping with daily pandemic life difficult. Many of my clients with pelvic/sexual pain also worry about whether they would survive COVID-19 or acquire long-COVID due to their health difficulties. For some, this fear may be overblown, but for those with immune issues and overall poor health, this concern is very real.

## Important Takeaways

- The experiences of a sexual trauma and having a pelvic/sexual pain disorder often share similar betrayal traumas.
- Clinicians must assess for all "layers of betrayal" to ensure trauma-informed care for both survivors of sexual trauma and women with pelvic/sexual pain disorders. The layers of betrayal include institutional betrayal, family betrayal, betrayal by peers, social/cultural betrayal, and spiritual betrayal.
- Betrayal trauma can occur within the medical system, creating delays in diagnosis and treatment, resulting in more negative outcomes for women with pelvic/sexual pain.
- Barriers that prevent women from receiving adequate healthcare include the cost of treatment and lack of health insurance coverage for pelvic/sexual pain disorders, lack of time and energy due to the burden of the "second shift," lack of physician education and

training regarding pelvic/sexual pain disorders, microaggressions or bias in the healthcare system, the development of a "learned helplessness" mindset after years of being dismissed by healthcare providers, and the unfolding impact of COVID-19.

# References

Bontempo, A. C., & Mikesell, L. (2020). Patient perceptions of misdiagnosis of endometriosis: Results from an online national survey. *Diagnosis*, 7(2), 97–106. https://doi.org/10.1515/dx-2019-0020

Carpenter, J. (2018, February 21). The unpaid work that always falls to women. *CNNMoney*. https://money.cnn.com/2018/02/21/pf/women-unpaid-work/index.html

Cleary, M. (2018, February 27). *Insurance 101: A guide on how to get your surgery covered*. Endometriosis: Causes – Symptoms – Diagnosis – and Treatment. www.endofound.org/insurance-101-a-guide-on-how-to-get-your-surgery-covered

Dickler, J. (2021, November 10). *Home prices are now rising much faster than incomes, studies show*. Retrieved November 14, 2021, from www.cnbc.com/2021/11/10/home-prices-are-now-rising-much-faster-than-incomes-studies-show.html

Eardley, I., Reisman, Y., Goldstein, S., Kramer, A., Dean, J., & Coleman, E. (2017). Existing and future educational needs in graduate and postgraduate education. *The Journal of Sexual Medicine*, 14(4), 475–485. https://doi.org/10.1016/j.jsxm.2017.01.014

Elbeshbishi, S. (2022, January 18). How sexual assault victims became incapacitated often decides charges. *USA Today*. Retrieved January 22, 2022, from www.usatoday.com/web-stories/how-sexual-assault-victims-became-incapacitated-often-decides-charges/

Evans, S., Dowding, C., Druitt, M., & Mikocka-Walus, A. (2021). "I'm in ISO all the time anyway": A mixed methods study on the impact of covid-19 on women with endometriosis. *Journal of Psychosomatic Research*, 146, 110508. https://doi.org/10.1016/j.jpsychores.2021.110508

Fairchild, P. S., Haefner, J. K., & Berger, M. B. (2016). Talk about sex: Sexual history-taking preferences among urogynecology patients and general gynecology controls. *Female Pelvic Medicine & Reconstructive Surgery*, 22(5), 297–302. https://doi.org/10.1097/spv.0000000000000291

Harlow, B. L., Wise, L. A., & Stewart, E. G. (2001). Prevalence and predictors of chronic lower genital tract discomfort. *American Journal of Obstetrics and Gynecology, 185*(3), 545–550. https://doi.org/10.1067/mob.2001.116748

Jacob, C. (2022, February 1). *Young people are increasingly overwhelmed at work, survey shows.* Retrieved February 03, 2022, from www.cnbc.com/2022/02/01/young-people-are-increasingly-overwhelmed-at-work-bain-co-survey.html

Kassebaum, N. J., Barber, R. M., Bhutta, Z. A., Dandona, L., Gething, P. W., Hay, S. I., Kinfu, Y., Larson, H. J., Liang, X., Lim, S. S., Lopez, A. D., Lozano, R., Mensah, G. A., Mokdad, A. H., Naghavi, M., Pinho, C., Salomon, J. A., Steiner, C., Vos, T., . . . Murray, C. J. (2016). Global, regional, and national levels of maternal mortality, 1990–2015: A systematic analysis for the global burden of disease study 2015. *The Lancet, 388*(10053), 1775–1812. https://doi.org/10.1016/s0140-6736(16)31470-2

Kingsberg, S. A., Schaffir, J., Faught, B. M., Pinkerton, J. A. V., Parish, S. J., Iglesia, C. B., Gudeman, J., Krop, J., & Simon, J. A. (2019). Female sexual health: Barriers to optimal outcomes and a roadmap for improved patient – clinician communications. *Journal of Women's Health, 28*(4), 432–443. https://doi.org/10.1089/jwh.2018.7352

Martínez-Zamora, M.-A., Coloma, J. L., Gracia, M., Rius, M., Castelo-Branco, C., & Carmona, F. (2021). Long-term follow-up of sexual quality of life after laparoscopic surgery in patients with deep infiltrating endometriosis. *Journal of Minimally Invasive Gynecology.* https://doi.org/10.1016/j.jmig.2021.04.023

Melillo, G. (2020, December 3). US ranks worst in maternal care, mortality compared with 10 other developed nations. *AJMC.* www.ajmc.com/view/us-ranks-worst-in-maternal-care-mortality-compared-with-10-other-developed-nations

Shindel, A. W., Baazeem, A., Eardley, I., & Coleman, E. (2016). Sexual health in undergraduate medical education: Existing and future needs and platforms. *The Journal of Sexual Medicine, 13*(7), 1013–1026. https://doi.org/10.1016/j.jsxm.2016.04.069

Smith, C. P., & Freyd, J. J. (2013). Dangerous safe havens: Institutional betrayal exacerbates sexual trauma. *Journal of Traumatic Stress, 26*(1), 119–124. doi:10.1002/jts.21778

Sue, D. W., & Spanierman, L. (2020). *Microaggressions in everyday life*. Wiley.

Worly, B., Manriquez, M., Stagg, A., Blanchard, M. H., Ogburn, T., Carson, S. A., & Woodland, M. B. (2021). Sexual health education in obstetrics and gynecology (Ob-Gyn) residencies – a resident physician survey. *The Journal of Sexual Medicine*, *18*(6), 1042–1052. https://doi.org/10.1016/j.jsxm.2021.03.005

# 5

## CULTURALLY COMPETENT ASSESSMENT FOR WOMEN WITH PELVIC/SEXUAL PAIN DISORDERS

DOI: 10.4324/9781003168232-5

## Assessment Overview

Assessment begins at the first point of contact, whether through email or phone call, when clients first reach out and explain why she is seeking therapy. After speaking with the client, if I am an appropriate fit for the client, an initial appointment is scheduled. If I determine during the initial contact that I am not the best fit for the client, I refer the client to a therapist who can better meet their needs. During the initial appointment, intake paperwork is reviewed, including the confidentiality contract and general practice policies. After these necessary steps are completed, I ask clients more about what is bringing them to therapy. I explain to clients that in our initial meeting, we can focus on the presenting problems and goals for therapy but that in the following few sessions, we will complete an extensive history as part of the assessment.

Especially with my pelvic/sexual pain clients, I inform them during the first session that they should let me know if they need to sit or lie in a more comfortable position due to pain. Some clients choose to bring special cushions or seats moving forward. During the first meeting, it is important to note the non-verbal communication of the client. For instance, a client may report they are in a significant amount of physical pain but have a very flat affect and are not expressing any physical signs of being in pain like fidgeting, grimacing, requesting to stand or lie down in session, crying, etc. This discrepancy could be the result of medications or dissociation or may be a sign that the client is having difficulty coping with even low levels of pain.

Clients vary in their comfort level in terms of what they share during the initial meeting. With openness and curiosity, I may gently ask questions, but I generally let the client go the direction they need during our first meeting. I like to establish what diagnoses they've had in the past and what their current diagnosis and treatment plan is. Most clients have multiple diagnoses and lack a treatment plan or treatment team.

During the following few sessions, I use the genogram as a tool to gather data in the next few sessions with the client (Bowen, 1978; Bowen, 1980; DeMaria et al., 2017; McGoldrick et al., 2008). Most of the sexually focused questions I use during my assessment are based on the work of Berman and Hof (1987), DeMaria et al. (1999), and Kaplan

(1983). However, I do ask more specific questions about pelvic/sexual pain disorders. I explain that the genogram is similar to a family tree, and it will help me to organize information about their family of origin. I show clients what I am drawing and adding to the genogram as the sessions progress. For examples of genograms for each of the vignettes, please see Figures 5.1 to 5.5.

While completing the assessment and creating the genogram, I collect information about the following four factors: medical/physiological factors, psychological factors, relational factors, and sociocultural factors. Important medical/physiological factors include current and past medications and treatments, history of any chronic illnesses or surgeries, disabilities or physical limitations, medical issues that were a direct result of a traumatic event, and a family history of medical issues. I ask for a detailed history of events one to two years before the onset of a chronic illness, including pelvic/sexual pain disorders. There may be life stressors or medical events leading up to the onset of the pelvic/sexual pain symptoms that likely contributed, but the client may be unaware of the connection. For instance, about a year and a half prior to experiencing pain with sex, one client had bariatric weight loss surgery, causing her to lose over 100 pounds. She explained she felt in the best shape of her life and felt more confident in dating, but now she was having pain with sex. As I had suspected, the pelvic floor physical therapist I referred the client to believed the rapid weight loss caused the client to develop pelvic floor muscle dysfunction.

It is important to assess with the client how these medical or physiological factors have impacted the way they view themselves as women and sexual beings. For instance, a client with endometriosis who was struggling to get pregnant due to the disease expressed feeling like a "failure" of a woman and wife. Prior to experiencing infertility, this client described herself as confident in her sexuality and as a woman and having always enjoyed sex. Infertility derailed her sexual self-esteem and was now also the driving force of her low sexual desire. Another reason information gathered about the medical/physiological factors are so important is that it helps clinicians to determine if the client currently has an appropriate treatment team. If the client lacks a treatment team, establishing an effective treatment team will likely become an early priority in treatment.

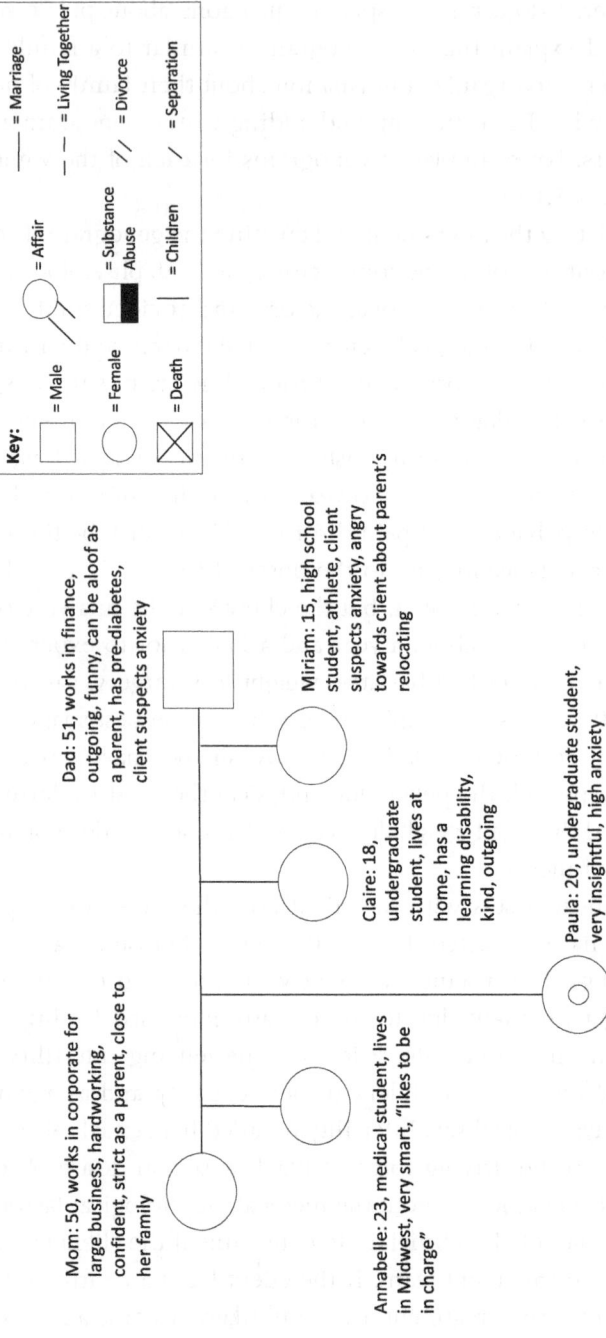

Presenting Problem: Paula reports painful intercourse and ongoing stress related to ongoing legal proceedings

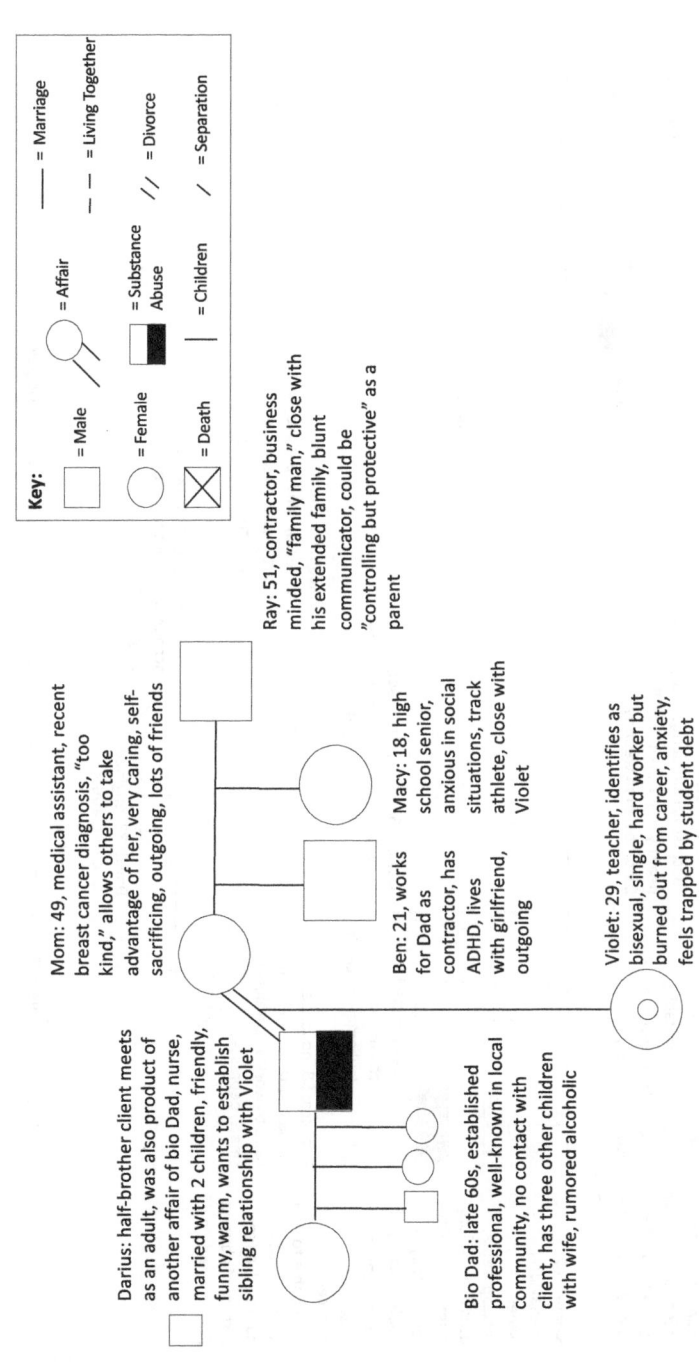

**Key:**

◻ = Male    ○⟋ = Affair    ——— = Marriage

○ = Female    ▨ = Substance Abuse    – – – = Living Together

⊠ = Death    | = Children    ⟋⟋ = Divorce

⟋ = Separation

Mom: 49, medical assistant, recent breast cancer diagnosis, "too kind," allows others to take advantage of her, very caring, self-sacrificing, outgoing, lots of friends

Ray: 51, contractor, business minded, "family man," close with his extended family, blunt communicator, could be "controlling but protective" as a parent

Darius: half-brother client meets as an adult, was also product of another affair of bio Dad, nurse, married with 2 children, friendly, funny, warm, wants to establish sibling relationship with Violet

Ben: 21, works for Dad as contractor, has ADHD, lives with girlfriend, outgoing

Macy: 18, high school senior, anxious in social situations, track athlete, close with Violet

Bio Dad: late 60s, established professional, well-known in local community, no contact with client, has three other children with wife, rumored alcoholic

Violet: 29, teacher, identifies as bisexual, single, hard worker but burned out from career, anxiety, feels trapped by student debt

Presenting Problem: Violet reports chronic pelvic pain and anxiety

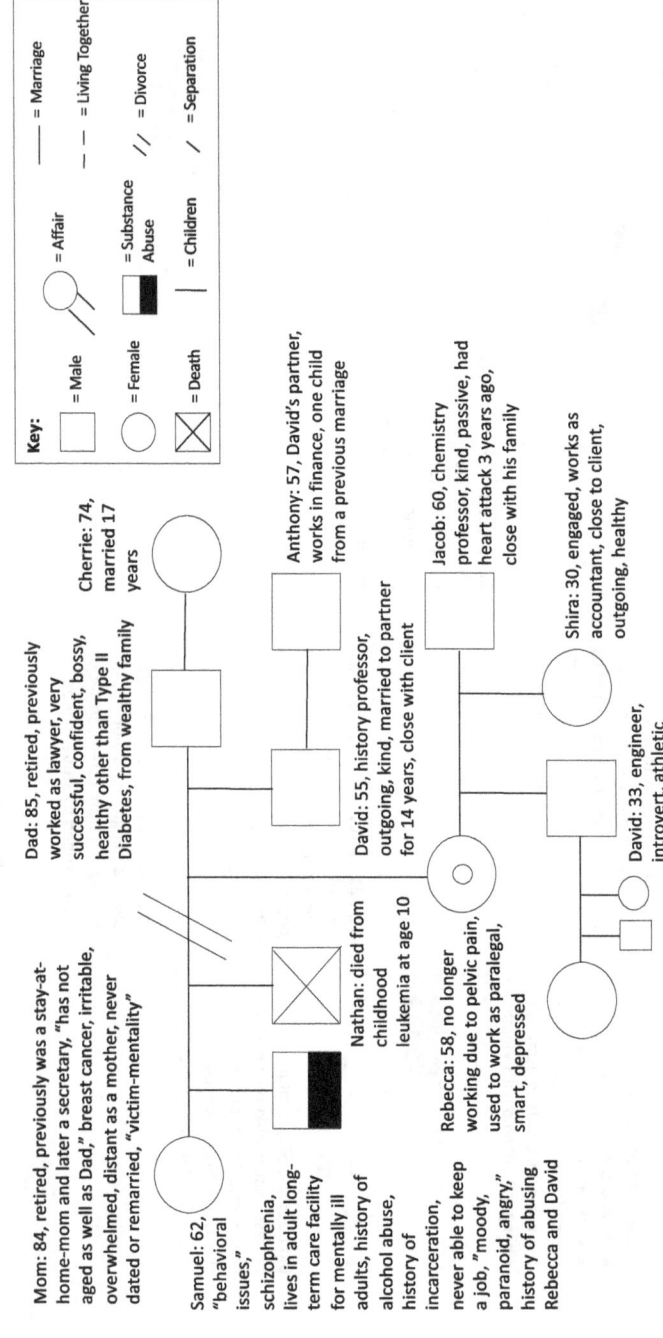

Key:

☐ = Male          ◯⟋ = Affair          ——— = Marriage

◯ = Female        ◨ = Substance Abuse   – – – = Living Together

⊠ = Death         | = Children          ⫽ = Divorce

                                        ⁄ = Separation

Cherrie: 74, married 17 years

Dad: 85, retired, previously worked as lawyer, very successful, confident, bossy, healthy other than Type II Diabetes, from wealthy family

Mom: 84, retired, previously was a stay-at-home-mom and later a secretary, "has not aged as well as Dad," breast cancer, irritable, overwhelmed, distant as a mother, never dated or remarried, "victim-mentality"

Anthony: 57, David's partner, works in finance, one child from a previous marriage

David: 55, history professor, outgoing, kind, married to partner for 14 years, close with client

Jacob: 60, chemistry professor, kind, passive, had heart attack 3 years ago, close with his family

Shira: 30, engaged, works as accountant, close to client, outgoing, healthy

Samuel: 62, "behavioral issues," schizophrenia, lives in adult long-term care facility for mentally ill adults, history of alcohol abuse, history of incarceration, never able to keep a job, "moody, paranoid, angry," history of abusing Rebecca and David

Nathan: died from childhood leukemia at age 10

Rebecca: 58, no longer working due to pelvic pain, used to work as paralegal, smart, depressed

David: 33, engineer, introvert, athletic

Presenting Problem: Rebecca reports anxiety and depression due to unresolved chronic pelvic pain

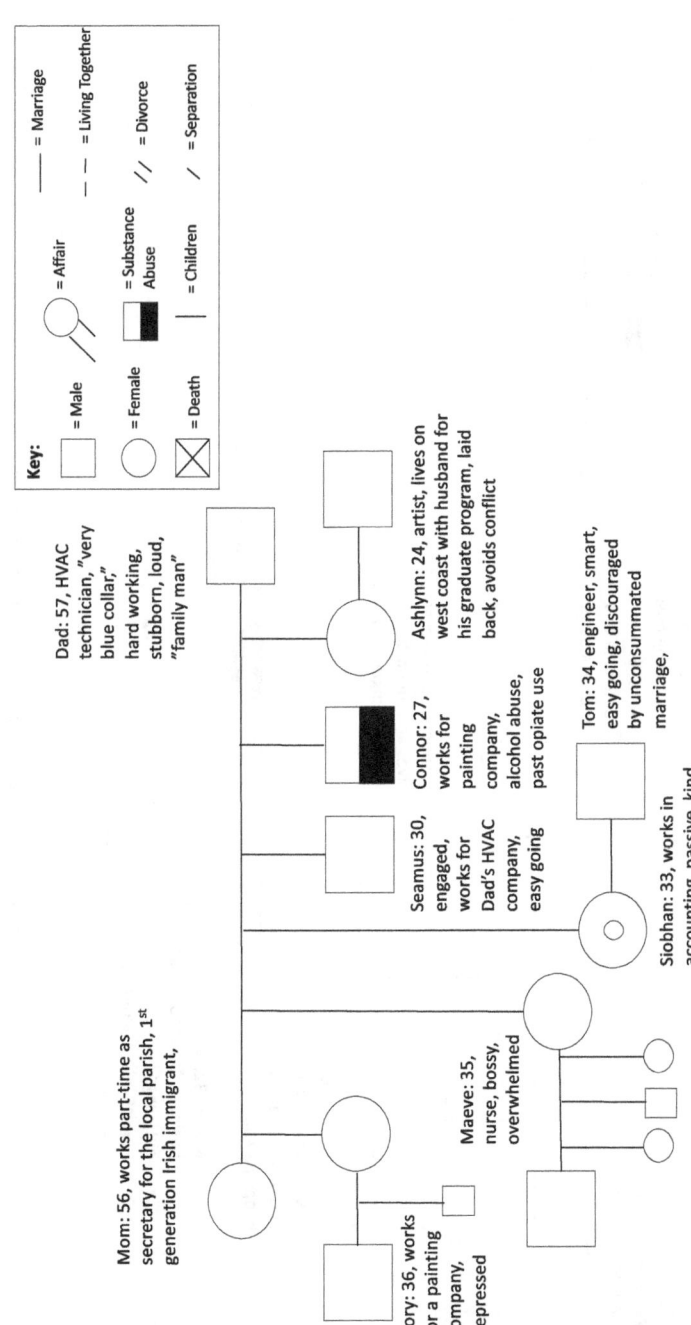

Key:

☐ = Male    ◯ = Female    ⊠ = Death

◯⟍ = Affair    ☐ (half-shaded) = Substance Abuse    | = Children

——— = Marriage    — — = Living Together    // = Divorce    / = Separation

Dad: 57, HVAC technician, "very blue collar," hard working, stubborn, loud, "family man"

Mom: 56, works part-time as secretary for the local parish, 1st generation Irish immigrant,

Seamus: 30, engaged, works for Dad's HVAC company, easy going

Connor: 27, works for painting company, alcohol abuse, past opiate use

Ashlynn: 24, artist, lives on west coast with husband for his graduate program, laid back, avoids conflict

Tom: 34, engineer, smart, easy going, discouraged by unconsummated marriage,

Siobhan: 33, works in accounting, passive, kind

Maeve: 35, nurse, bossy, overwhelmed

Rory: 36, works for a painting company, depressed

Presenting Problem: Siobhan reports being unable to have penetrative sex with husband

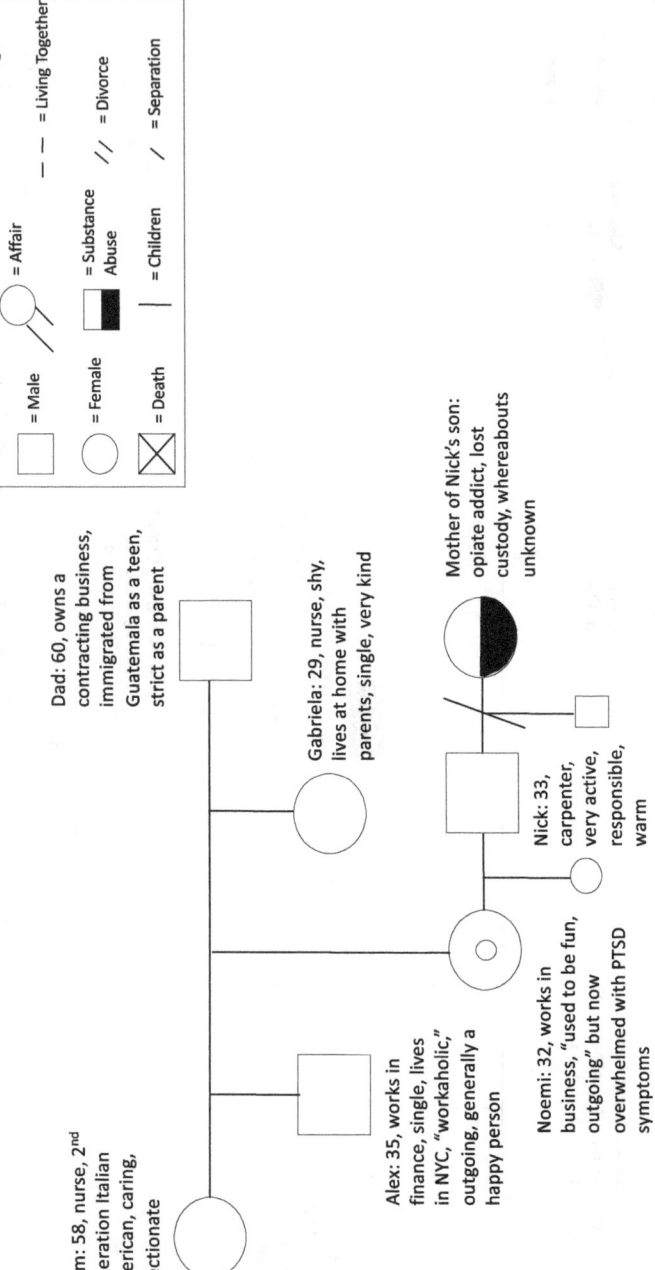

**Key:**

□ = Male

○ = Female

⊠ = Death

○⌐ = Affair

▣ = Substance Abuse

⊢ = Children

——— = Marriage

– – – = Living Together

// = Divorce

/ = Separation

Mom: 58, nurse, 2nd generation Italian American, caring, affectionate

Dad: 60, owns a contracting business, immigrated from Guatemala as a teen, strict as a parent

Gabriela: 29, nurse, shy, lives at home with parents, single, very kind

Mother of Nick's son: opiate addict, lost custody, whereabouts unknown

Nick: 33, carpenter, very active, responsible, warm

Alex: 35, works in finance, single, lives in NYC, "workaholic," outgoing, generally a happy person

Noemi: 32, works in business, "used to be fun, outgoing" but now overwhelmed with PTSD symptoms

Presenting Problem: Noemi reports PTSD symptoms and painful sex

Psychological factors include the client's history of psychotherapy or psychiatric care, history of any diagnoses and medications, family history of mental health and substance abuse issues, the strengths and resources available to address psychological issues, and barriers to addressing psychological issues. Consider the ways these psychological factors have impacted the client's life and the way she views herself sexually. One client expressed high levels of shame around hypersexual behavior during manic episodes prior to being diagnosed and medicated for bipolar disorder. Now dealing with a painful sex, the feelings of shame became even more overwhelming, making it difficult for her to want to engage sexually with her partner.

Make note of "big T" and "little t traumas" over the course of the client's life and if mental health issues emerged around these time periods. Women are often misdiagnosed, especially those with trauma histories. For women with a mental health diagnosis, I ask if they believe the diagnosis fits. I often find my trauma clients wondering if their symptoms are posttraumatic stress disorder (PTSD) rather than a mood disorder or personality disorder. Referral to a psychiatrist is useful for clients who question their diagnosis or do not find their current medications helpful. Common co-occurring diagnoses I often see with pelvic/sexual pain disorders include generalized anxiety disorder, major depressive disorder, obsessive-compulsive disorder, and PTSD. Patients with pelvic/sexual pain disorders, even in those with mental illness, can be successfully treated; however, the mental illness must be prioritized in treatment, especially if it is a significant barrier to a client's ability to engage in treatment.

Relational history includes information about important relationships, including the family of origin, romantic partners, and close friends. Obtain basic information about immediate family – parents, siblings, partners, children, or any other important extended family member – including those who have lived or live in the client's home. I gather the following information about each family member: (1) age; (2) if they have passed away, when and what were the cause of death; (3) current and past employment; (4) any medical or mental health issues; and (5) how the client would describe this family member's personality in a sentence of two. Ask about the client's role in their family of origin and how they believe others in their family view them. I also like to know who they were close to in their family growing up versus as an adult.

Make sure to gather information about the client's past and current partners, including the length of relationships and why the relationships ended. Clients who have been dealing with their pelvic/sexual pain condition since their teen or young adult years may note significant impacts to their dating and relationship history. For those in long-term partnerships, it is important to note at what point did the pelvic/sexual pain symptoms appeared and when they became an issue for the couple.

I typically ask about their first sexual experiences while gathering the information related to relational factors. It is also important to note the messages the client was exposed to regarding gender roles, especially those related to sex and sexuality. Because most sexual abuse is perpetrated by someone the victim knows, it is important to look for possible patterns of abuse in the family. A client may not be ready to disclose abuse that happened within the family system during the assessment, so make sure to look out for red flags of grooming behavior by family members or other adults that were close to the client. Note how the family attitudes and beliefs have impacted the way the client views herself as a woman and views her body, her sexuality, and even her pelvic/sexual pain. Lack of support and negative attitudes of family members about the client's symptoms can exacerbate the client's distress.

When assessing for sociocultural factors make sure to consider the varying influences across the client's development. Sociocultural factors include race, culture, ethnicity, religion, and even socioeconomic status. Discuss with the client how sociocultural attitudes and beliefs have impacted the way they view themselves as women, their bodies, their sexuality, and their pelvic/sexual pain. Sociocultural factors should be always assessed for during each phase of the assessment, thus interweaving questions regarding sociocultural factors throughout the assessment process. Clinicians must demonstrate cultural competence while assessing for the impact of sociocultural factors.

Lee and Park (2013) explain that a culturally competent therapist has "awareness, knowledge, and skills to intervene effectively" with clients from diverse backgrounds (p. 6). Lee (2013) also contends that a culturally competent therapist "simultaneously acknowledges human similarity and celebrates human difference" (p. 17). Lee (2015) explains that therapists often view a client's culture as an external factor rather than something internalized or psychological. Therapists who believe culture is an external factor often think understanding the client's cultural background will automatically lead to insight about the client, which is obviously not the case. Ho (1995) coined the term "internalized culture" and argues that culture is a psychological construct instead of an anthropologic construct. Ho defined "internalized culture" as "the cultural influences operating inside the individual that share (not determine) personality formation and various aspects of psychological functioning" (p. 5).

In tune with the consensus in our field, I believe cultural competence is necessary in understanding the role of factors, including culture, ethnicity, race, disability status, religion, sexual orientation, gender orientation, and experiences of discrimination, in our clients' lives. The ability to understand these factors will help you to join with the client and will contribute to a more accurate assessment (Lee & Park, 2013; Moodley et al., 2015; Sue & Sue, 2015). The more accurate and culturally attuned the assessment, the more likely you will be able to establish appropriate treatment goals with the client that consider their values and real-life barriers.

## Important Assessment Questions

I enjoy approaching the assessment phase of treatment with openness and curiosity. Clinicians must be able to ask difficult questions sometimes while remaining in tune with the client's boundaries and comfort level regarding sharing, especially early in treatment. Learning when to probe further versus deciding to circle back to a question at a later point is a skill therapists develop over years. I have found this skill invaluable with my pelvic/sexual pain clients and those with traumatic experiences, who often enter therapy struggling to make sense of their story. While the questions provided next are not an exhaustive list, I have found these assessment questions particularly significant for women presenting with pelvic/sexual pain. For each question, I provide an example of dialogue between myself, the therapist, and one of the clients from the case vignettes.

### How Long have You Had Pelvic/Sexual Pain Symptoms?

In most cases, women with pelvic/sexual pain disorders have been living with the symptoms for years. It is useful to know the amount of time the client has been experiencing symptoms because the negative impact on the client's life is likely to be more significant the longer they have contended with symptoms.

THERAPIST: How long have you been experiencing these symptoms?

VIOLET: Heavy and painful periods started for me pretty much shortly after I got my period at 13. I had pain with sex, deep pain, with my high school boyfriend. I thought since it was my first time that maybe it was normal, but then it continued. By the time I was in graduate school, my symptoms were severe.

THERAPIST: It seems like these symptoms have evolved over time. What were the most distressing symptoms for you in graduate school?

VIOLET: The pain was terrible, but the thing that interfered most with my ability to get on with my day was the vomiting and very heavy bleeding when I would get my period. I basically couldn't do anything for about a week.

THERAPIST: That's awful. How did you get through school while dealing with that?

VIOLET: Not well. I did miss quite a few days of classes when I would get my period. I didn't feel like I could say to my professors, "I'm missing class because I have my period" [laughs]. The absences did lower my grades.

THERAPIST: Tell me about your symptoms currently.

VIOLET: Some of my symptoms did improve after the surgery, and now I take the pill continuously, which I think has helped a lot. Currently, though, I have a lot of bladder pressure and feeling like I need to pee and [have] general pelvic pain; basically, that whole region can be painful sometimes. I also have a lot of fatigue. Sometimes I can wake up, go on a walk, and then be ready for a nap by ten in the morning. Maybe it's not related to my endometriosis, and it is burnout related? Either way, it's an issue for sure.

THERAPIST: What about painful sex? Has that still been an issue?

VIOLET: Funny you ask because I was thinking about that because I knew I had this appointment coming up. Basically, I don't know [laughs]. I haven't had penetrative sex in a few years, and I haven't really been dating in general the last two-ish years. My most recent partner was a woman, and we didn't have penetrative sex.

THERAPIST: Okay. . . . Were you able to have pleasurable sex with your most recent partner?

VIOLET: Yes, totally. But for sure, my symptoms got in the way of having the energy or desire to engage sometimes.

## How Did You Come to be Diagnosed With your Pelvic/Sexual Pain Disorder?

These are usually long and painful stories for clients to recount. Some clients are eager to share their journey with someone who is wanting to listen, while others need time to unpack their story more slowly and over multiple sessions. Ideally in the first session, you at least want to know the age at which they began to experience symptoms, their most distressing symptoms, past and current diagnoses, and the ages at which they received these diagnoses. Many women will also explain that they either do not have a diagnosis currently or that they believe their current diagnosis is incorrect. It is very important to pay attention to the emotions these stories evoke. If a client appears flat, it may be from high doses of medications, such as gabapentin, or it could reflect how emotionally shut down they are. Others may be highly emotional and struggle with regulation. If a client seems highly depressed or anxious, you should also screen for suicidality.

THERAPIST: How did you get the diagnosis of vulvodynia?

SIOBHAN: I went to my first gynecology appointment when I was 30 because I was worried about something being wrong. We'd been married for two years and were still not having sex.

THERAPIST: Okay, but do you know why the doctor thought you had vulvodynia?

SIOBHAN: I guess because I said the exam was really painful? I jumped off the table!

THERAPIST: The pain must have been really bad. Do you remember where the pain was?

SIOBHAN: Honestly, no. The doctor barely touched me, and I just felt that panic again and jumped off the table. I googled vulvodynia after that, but I don't think it fits me. Then I found vaginismus when I was searching and thought wow, that sounds like me.

### Who is a Part of your Current Treatment Team?

Do not be surprised if you hear the response, "I don't have a treatment team." Many women with pelvic/sexual pain conditions are passed from specialist to specialist over years. Others have grown so frustrated with their experiences in the healthcare system that they stop seeking help. Some clients may have one or two providers on their treatment team. Identifying who is a part of the treatment will inform you about what other healthcare providers you need to connect with to ensure collaborative care. Clinicians will also be able to determine gaps in the client's treatment team and where the client may need to add healthcare providers.

THERAPIST: Who is part of your current treatment team?

NOEMI: Well . . . [laughs] you? That's it.

THERAPIST: [laughs] Sadly, that's usually the norm. But we're going to make sure you have others on your treatment team for sure. First, I think we need to help you with your trauma symptoms, and then we can figure out who else you should see to treat your pelvic pain.

NOEMI: My OB/GYN does know a little bit about what is going on. She did encourage me to go to counseling, but she was thinking most of this is postpartum related.

THERAPIST: Okay – good. Has she been able to help regarding painful sex?

NOEMI: Honestly . . . no? I think her intentions are good, but she basically just told me to use a lot of lube and have a glass of wine. She also said that this was just sex after having a baby. But I don't think this is normal.

### What is Your Current Treatment Plan?

Again, do not be surprised if you hear the response, "I don't have a treatment plan." Some women may have received initial care but did not continue with their treatment plan. This is often the result of women facing multiple barriers, including financial constraints, feeling ignored by their healthcare providers, being time poor, etc. If the client does have a treatment plan, it is important to know what the plan entails, including medications, injections, physical therapy, etc.

You should know the frequency of treatments and dosage of medications. Make sure to ask the client's opinion on their treatment plan. To what extent do they believe their treatment plan has helped them? I also like to know if they believe there are any gaps in their treatment plan. To get a description for baseline symptoms versus a flare-up of symptoms, you can use a 0 to 10 scale, where 0 is no pain at all and 10 is pain so severe you need to go to the emergency room.

THERAPIST: What is your current treatment plan for your endometriosis and pelvic pain?

VIOLET: Since my surgery, I have just been doing oral birth control continuously.

THERAPIST: Who is prescribing that for you?

VIOLET: My regular gynecologist.

THERAPIST: Do you think that has been helping?

VIOLET: It's helping because I rarely get my period now, but obviously, it's not going to make the endometriosis go away.

THERAPIST: Did the surgeon or your regular gynecologist suggest any other forms of treatment?

VIOLET: At my postop, we talked about Lupron, which I really don't want to do because of the side effects. Other than that, no.

THERAPIST: On a 0 to 10 scale, where 0 is no pain at all and 10 is pain so severe you need to go to the emergency room, where would you rate your daily baseline of symptoms? What about a flare-up of your symptoms?

VIOLET: I might have to think about that more . . . but offhand, baseline maybe a 3 or 4? But when I am in a flare-up, probably about an 8.

THERAPIST: And how often would you say you're in a flare-up?

VIOLET: Since the surgery and since being on the pill continuously, it's been less, but maybe still once a month for a few days I feel worse.

### What Have You Tried in the Past to Treat Your Pelvic/Sexual Pain Disorder?

It is important to know what clients have tried in the past and whether these treatments were successful or not. It is important to know for how long the client tried each intervention. For instance, a client may tell you that pelvic floor physical therapy did not help them, but if they only attended five appointments, it would be unlikely that they would notice any improvements. This information may point the clinician to the types of specialists the client may currently need. It can also help the clinician detect possible signs of psychological factors interfering with treatment progress.

THERAPIST: What have you tried before to treat your pelvic pain?

REBECCA: What *haven't* I tried? [sarcastically]

THERAPIST: It would be helpful for me to know.

REBECCA: [long sigh] Well . . . I've done about 3 years of pelvic floor physical therapy, I've done a few rounds of nerve blocks, I've tried all kinds of injections and creams, I've tried antidepressants and some other pain medications, and I'm probably forgetting a few other things. . . . Oh – hypnosis. My husband wanted me to try that one because his colleague's wife thought it worked for arthritis pain.

THERAPIST: Of everything you have tried, what has helped the most?

REBECCA: That's difficult to answer . . . because nothing has helped that much. The nerve blocks always did give me at least a little temporary relief. Physical therapy just seems to flare everything back up, but I continue to torture myself with that. I had a lot of side effects to the medications, and I didn't feel as though they helped very much, so I stopped those. Hypnosis was a joke. Not sure where Jacob found that woman. Complete whack-a-doo.

THERAPIST: You've tried a lot of different treatments. It must be frustrating to feel like nothing has helped.

REBECCA: [tearful] Yes. I really have tried a lot but with little success.

THERAPIST: Your physical therapist . . . you've worked with her now for three years. Have the two of you discussed why you may not be responding to treatments as hoped?

REBECCA: We have talked about it, and it's part of why she referred me to you. She's been wondering if maybe I have "complex regional pain syndrome" or that maybe my nervous system is overactive . . . which who knows, maybe.

### Are You Taking Any Medications?

Always obtain a full account of past and current medication. Pay close attention to who is prescribing the different medications. Because some women have so many different healthcare providers, they may be on medications that should not be combined with one another or are negating the effect of the other. Many women who have pelvic/sexual pain are prescribed high levels of gabapentin or amitriptyline, which can cause flat affect, slow cognition, fatigue, depression, and constipation, which can worsen pelvic floor symptoms. Also be wary of women who have been prescribed opioids for daily pain relief. Even when prescribed by a doctor, the client could be addicted. Many women with pelvic/sexual pain disorders also present with low sexual desire. It is important to know whether clients are taking selective serotonin reuptake inhibitors, which can cause or exacerbate low libido. You may find that other clients have been prescribed medication but either never filled them or never used them. If this is the case, ask why they decided to not take the medication.

THERAPIST: Are you on any medication currently?

NOEMI: My primary care doctor put me on Zoloft because she thinks I have postpartum depression.

THERAPIST: How do you feel the Zoloft is working for you?

NOEMI: I thought maybe initially it was helping, but honestly, I don't know now. It's been a few months, but I still feel really irritable and angry. I still think about the birth trauma a lot. I've thought about going off it but wanted to see what you thought first.

THERAPIST: I can't prescribe medication, but I can refer you to a psychiatrist who specializes in maternal mental health. I think it's worth getting another opinion. If these symptoms are driven more by your trauma, then you might need a different medication.

NOEMI: Okay. At this point, I am open to seeing the psychiatrist.

THERAPIST: In the past, have you ever taken any other medications?

NOEMI: Well, I've never tried an antidepressant before Zoloft. After the hemorrhage, I was on iron pills for a few months. Other than that, I have taken an albuterol inhaler since I was a kid for occasional asthma issues.

### What Have Been the Most Difficult Parts of Having a Pelvic/Sexual Pain Disorder for You?

You want to understand the most difficult aspects of having a pelvic/sexual pain disorder for the client. For some, the most difficult parts are the impact on their sexuality and ability to connect intimately with a partner. For others, it is living with chronic pain or feeling different from others their age. Knowing the most difficult parts will help you to determine the more immediate therapeutic goals.

THERAPIST: What has been the hardest thing about having pelvic pain?

PAULA: I just want to be a normal college student, and having pain with sex is just this huge reminder that I'm not. I already feel different having to deal with this trial while going to school.

THERAPIST: I'm sorry. So, it's isolating, and it sounds like it's also a reminder of these other big stressors in your life.

PAULA: Definitely. Just makes me feel like in general, there is something wrong with me. Almost like I'm cursed or something.

### Tell Me About How Your Pelvic/Sexual Pain Condition Impacts your Daily Life

Even for clients with mild symptoms, the impact to daily life could be significant. Clinicians should understand how each client experiences the impact of their pelvic/sexual pain condition. Clinicians may be surprised at the level of limitations some clients live with, whether self-imposed or because of a healthcare professional's recommendation. Some clients might focus on the logistical issues, such as difficulty engaging in habits that will foster a healthy pelvic floor at work. Others note the significant emotional toll and isolation from others. Knowing the extent to which a client believes their daily life is impacted by their pelvic/sexual pain condition will allow you to create relevant goals with the client and help you to determine the therapeutic starting point.

THERAPIST: Tell me about how your daily life has been impacted by your pelvic pain.

REBECCA: It's impacted everything [tearful]. This forced me to retire, and even though I'm not working, I'm no use to my son. I can't even help with my grandchildren because I am so limited right now in what I am able to do. My daughter is getting married next summer, and I don't even think I would be able to go wedding dress shopping with her.

THERAPIST: Okay. Can you explain more about why that is? What becomes a barrier, for instance, in the wedding dress shopping example.

REBECCA: Well, first, I can't drive. My husband has basically become my "transporter." He has to put the back seats down because I cannot sit for longer than 15 to 20 minutes. So, I just lie down in the back of the car while he drives. Even if I could physically get to the wedding dress shop, I wouldn't be able to sit through the appointment. I'd have to get up every few minutes, probably lie down at some point, which is not okay to do in a store. I can't walk very far either, so I wouldn't be able to walk around and help my daughter pick out dresses. I also have to wear these super loose, awful sweatpants all of the time. I can't be in a shop with my daughter and her friends, with everyone dressed nice, and I look like I'm lying around in pajamas.

THERAPIST: Geez, the logistics of driving and trying to balance the sitting and standing is probably a big barrier to a lot of activities.

REBECCA: It's a huge issue!

THERAPIST: In terms of walking, has your physical therapist advised you not to walk very far?

REBECCA: No . . . but I notice my symptoms get so much worse if I walk, so I've been trying to limit my walking.

THERAPIST: How far would you say you walk in a day? Or how many steps?

REBECCA: I don't have a smart watch to count steps, so I don't know about steps, but I try not to walk more than a few minutes, a few times, each day.

THERAPIST: That sounds pretty restrictive.

REBECCA: It is, and especially when you compare it to how active I used to be. I used to go on 10, 11, 12, whatever mile hikes with my husband. Now I can hardly walk to the end of the driveway to get our mail.

THERAPIST: Tell me, what can you still do that brings you some joy?

REBECCA: The things that have always brought me the biggest joy have been outdoor activities. I have always hated being stuck in the house. . . . I think it reminds me of my childhood. So, right now, there isn't much. I like reading and sitting with my dogs. That's about it.

### What is the Story You Tell Yourself About Your Pelvic/Sexual Pain?

The client's response to this question often indicates the depth of the work that needs to be done. Responses that include shame, guilt, and blame usually mean deeper therapeutic work is warranted. One client told me she believed she was being "punished" by God for having an abortion as a young adult. Another client, who struggled with some physical challenges as a young child, told me her body had always "failed" her, and the pain with sex was simply just one more way she was "defective." Other clients may appear despondent or hopeless, usually due to years of suffering with a pelvic/sexual pain condition. One client explained that she believed it was simply her bad luck in life and that she did not expect her condition to improve at all. Some clients respond with high anxiety. As one client explained, she was not sure what was happening to her body and felt completely out of control. For Paula, the question elicited her intense feelings of shame about having been a victim of grooming-type abuse:

THERAPIST: What's the story you tell yourself about your pelvic/sexual pain?

PAULA: The story . . . like why am I having the pain?

THERAPIST: Yes, what do you tell yourself about that?

PAULA: I think my pain with sex is a big reminder of this big mistake I made. Huge mistake for sure. And also, the pain is just another reminder of what he has ruined for me. He has tainted me.

THERAPIST: So, when you experience the pain, is that what you think about?

PAULA: Pretty much. I guess the story is that I'm damaged goods.

### What Else Do These Feelings [Elicited by the Pelvic/Sexual Pain] Remind You of?

This question will help you determine if some of the strong feelings evoked by the pelvic/sexual pain condition have come up in reaction to another past experience, like a sexual trauma, for instance. If so, the shared emotional experiences could be triggering each other. Consider Noemi's response to this question:

THERAPIST: You've talked about how the pain with sex is making you feel powerless and out of control. Do those feelings remind you of anything else?

NOEMI: It does. I've told you that I was sexually assaulted at work right after college. Those are the same feelings I had after it happened.

THERAPIST: Powerless and out of control?

NOEMI: Yes, and also confused. Which I feel confused now too. I couldn't understand then why that was happening to me, and now I don't understand why my body is doing this.

THERAPIST: That makes sense.

NOEMI: Feeling confused . . . that also reminds me of the postpartum hemorrhage . . . it was sort of that same disbelief of how is this happening to me, and being confused too about what was actually happening with my body. For sure, in the hospital, I felt totally powerless and out of control, and I was. I went in and then woke up without a uterus.

### How Did You Learn About Sex?

For women who were raised in a more conservative environment where sex is viewed as a taboo subject, it is common to have developed guilt-related inhibitions or avoidance that could be exacerbating the pelvic/sexual pain disorder. Other women may have been raised in environments where they may have been exposed to sexual knowledge too young or sex was discussed in inappropriate ways, like, for example, inappropriate jokes or making sexually seductive comments.

THERAPIST: Do you remember how you learned about sex?

SIOBHAN: I don't know. I remember listening to some of my friends in high school talk about sex, but I don't know if I actually knew logistically what that meant. I knew that's how you had a baby. That's about it.

THERAPIST: Did your parents ever talk to you about sex?

SIOBHAN: The only time they talked about it was to tell me it was for marriage.

THERAPIST: Do you remember anything else about that conversation? What sparked it, perhaps?

SIOBHAN: Oh! I remember what sparked it [laughs]. My older brother Rory got his girlfriend pregnant in college. Huge family drama. My parents basically told him he had to marry her, so they had "shotgun wedding." Her parents wanted the marriage, too, since they are an extremely Catholic family. My parents were always worried after that about one of us getting pregnant.

THERAPIST: What about once you were ready to get married . . . was there any discussion about sex?

SIOBHAN: No, not really. I knew by that point the logistics of sex – I must have learned about this through friends, and I did some googling on my own.

### When Was Your First Sexual Experience, and How Did You Experience This? Positive? Neutral? Negative?

Some clients may respond to this question by asking, "What do you mean by sexual experience?" I often explain that it is the first experience they consider to be sexual. For some clients, it might be a first kiss, while for others, it may mean outercourse or penetrative sex. It is normal for clients who come from more conservative or religious backgrounds to not have had sexual experiences until marriage. Clients with lifelong vaginismus may have had little or no experiences that they identify as sexual. Many people, not just those with pelvic/sexual pain conditions, may have felt awkward or embarrassed by these first experiences. In addition, these experiences may not have always been consensual.

Once a client tells me a bit about their first sexual experience, if I need more information, I often ask, "Would you say it was a positive, neutral, or negative experience?" Sometimes this gives clients enough space to tell me if there was a coercive sexual experience or traumatic experience. I allow clients to tell me what they are comfortable with. If I feel like I need more information, I might ask, "Are you comfortable if I ask you a few more questions about that, or we can shelve this topic for later. Whatever you are most comfortable with right now."

THERAPIST: Tell me about your first sexual experience.

VIOLET: Intercourse or anything sexual?

THERAPIST: Either/or. Whatever you consider to be your first sexual experience.

VIOLET: My first sexual experience was in ninth grade, playing seven minutes in heaven at a party. It was very PG, maybe some second base going on, totally consensual. It was with one of my guy friends from school. The first time I had actual sex was with my boyfriend Jeff.

THERAPIST: What was your first experience with penetrative sex like?

VIOLET: Eh — it was okay.

THERAPIST: Why just okay?

VIOLET: For one thing, we had no idea what we were doing. We also always had to do it sneakily, like in Jeff's basement, so I was always worried about getting caught by his parents. And I did notice some pain.

## Have You Ever Had an Unwanted Sexual Experience?

I ask this question specifically in this way because some clients may not know how to label their experiences. Using the broader term "unwanted" gives many women who are struggling with their experiences the space to talk about these incidents without necessarily needing to categorize their experiences as assault, abuse, coercive, etc. Unwanted sexual experiences could include anything from a client walking in on their parents having sex, being exposed to porn accidently at a young age, being sexually harassed by a peer at school, or a teacher making inappropriate sexual comments towards them.

THERAPIST: Have you ever had any unwanted sexual experiences?

VIOLET: Yeah, in college. I was drinking with friends, and one of my guy friends invited me back to his room. We hung out alone before and never did anything together, so I didn't think he wanted to hook up or anything. We would usually just watch a movie and drunk munch on snacks for a while. But he tried to kiss me in his room, and I said no, and then he just kept going. I honestly don't even remember everything. But I don't think there was penetration. I think I got out of there before that happened. But he was kissing me and removing my clothes and touching me even though I kept telling him no.

THERAPIST: That's scary.

VIOLET: It was, and I don't really know what to call it either. I guess technically it is a sexual assault? Regardless, it was unwanted for sure. . . . The neighborhood I lived in during graduate school was a little rough. For sure there was some catcalling, and one time a guy grabbed my butt and followed me for a while. I thought that had the potential to end very badly. There were a lot of people around, but he still continued to follow me. I eventually went into a store and called the cops.

### Have You Been in a Long-Term Relationship Before? If So, How and Why Did the Relationship End?

It is always important to understand our clients' relationship histories and patterns. For women with pelvic/sexual pain disorders, it is important to understand the story they may be telling themselves about how their condition has impacted their dating histories – whether it is true or steeped in cognitive distortions. One young woman blamed her pelvic/sexual pain disorder for her long history of relationships ending after one or two months. However, upon exploration, she may have contributed to these relationships' failures with her own self-sabotage, which included avoiding all intimate contact and refusing to invite partners to her apartment or going to their homes. She also never disclosed to any of her partners that she had a pelvic/sexual pain disorder. Many of these partners told her when breaking up that they believed she was not interested in having a relationship, which was understandable given her behavior.

THERAPIST: You've told me that you're currently single but tell me about your dating history.

VIOLET: My first boyfriend was in high school. We dated for about a year. It was just sort of a sweet first love kind of thing. We broke up the summer before starting college; it was mutual, but it still sucked. We actually still stay in touch, and I would say we're friends. He's married now.

THERAPIST: What about in college?

VIOLET: That was sort of a confusing time for me. I was questioning my sexuality more and really did want to date women but had no clue how to navigate that. I mostly hooked up in college, usually with guys, but did not have sex with most of these hook-ups. I was having pain with sex pretty bad at that point, so penetrative sex didn't have a huge appeal to me. Which, actually, I think made me doubt my own interest in women. I remember thinking, "Well, maybe you only think you like women because you're just trying to avoid sex." I did kiss a few girls in college, but that feels so stereotypical.

THERAPIST: Were you able to date women later? Especially since that was an experience you were wanting.

VIOLET: After college while I was still in Tennessee, no. But I wasn't dating anyone. I think I was just really preoccupied with my next steps, and honestly, my health was not in a good place. But during graduate school I did. The dating scene for women dating women was much better, obviously, in a big East Coast city. I finally started to meet other women who didn't scoff at me identifying as bisexual. I dated one woman, Alicia, for about a year. We were about to move in together, which was even her idea, but she bailed. It was pretty painful, and I didn't really get an explanation. She sent me a vague email about a month later saying she needed to "find herself" and that she felt like she let the relationship become her whole identity. Worst break-up of my life.

THERAPIST: Where are you emotionally with that break-up now?

VIOLET: Even though it's been a few years, honestly, I'm pretty bitter about it. I think it's made it harder for me to get back out there. Like I've dated since then but pretty casually. And now with knowing for sure that I can't have kids, I just feel like it's another barrier to finding a long-term partner.

### Tell Me About Your Partner

If a client is partnered, it is helpful to learn more about their current relationship. Of importance is to know whether the partner is aware of the pelvic/sexual pain disorder. In addition, it is important to know if the client entered the relationship already having had the pelvic/sexual pain disorder or if the onset occurred during the course of the relationship.

THERAPIST: Tell me about how you met Tom.

SIOBHAN: I met Tom when I was 26 at my friend's Christmas party.

THERAPIST: How did you guys end up dating?

SIOBHAN: He got my number from one of my friends after the party. I thought he was cute, so when he did call, I agreed to go out on a date with him.

THERAPIST: What do you like about Tom?

SIOBHAN: We have similar upbringings and values. He is very smart and loyal. We usually have fun together.

THERAPIST: When did you guys decide to get married?

SIOBHAN: We were pretty serious from the beginning. He was waiting to have sex for marriage, too. We dated for one year, then were engaged for a year and got married.

THERAPIST: When did you both learn about the vaginismus?

SIOBHAN: I always suspected something was wrong, but I don't know why. I guess we both figured out on our honeymoon when we couldn't have sex. We tried lots of times.

THERAPIST: What do you mean you guys tried?

SIOBHAN: We would be in bed kissing, and I knew he wanted to have sex, but I would just get sort of panicked.

THERAPIST: Okay – so did he ever try to penetrate you? Or did things never progress that far?

SIOBHAN: I've never even taken my underwear off, so no, things never progressed that far. And I think we both thought with time, the sex thing would get easier, or I would get less anxious, but that obviously hasn't happened in five years.

### How Supportive is Your Partner in Towards Your Pelvic/Sexual Pain Disorder?

This question is imperative for any client who is partnered and will tell you more about the possible relationship support and distress caused by the pelvic/sexual pain disorder. Many partners are supportive of the client with pelvic/sexual pain. Supportive behavior from partners may look like focusing on pleasurable sexual activities rather than penetrative sexual activities. It also looks like the partner prioritizing the client's treatment, including doctor's appointments, pelvic floor physical therapy, dilator therapy and counseling. Even those with supportive partners may fear that their partners will still leave without enough sexual contact, which may highlight some of their own insecurities rather than the partners'. Some women may claim their partners are supportive, but they fail to step up in terms of sharing the childcare or the household burden, which would enable the client to make time for treatment. I have also unfortunately seen many cases when a client continues to engage in very painful penetrative sexual activities due to intense pressure from the partner or their own fears that the partner will have an affair or leave the relationship. Sometimes these sexual encounters are coercive or abusive, and clients struggle with how to label their own participation.

THERAPIST: Has Parker been supportive of you getting treatment for your pelvic pain?

PAULA: Oh, yeah. He knows I'm here, and from the first time I told him, he said I should see a doctor. And I didn't tell him right away; I was sort of suffering through sex for a while. He kept asking me what was wrong, and I think he thought he was doing something wrong.

THERAPIST: Once you told him, did you guys adjust what you've been doing sexually?

PAULA: We don't have sex right now. Not until I can get everything figured out. But we do other things, but I am comfortable with those. [tearing up] I worry he's going to leave me because we're not having sex.

THERAPIST: Has he ever said that he will leave? Or indicated he will?

PAULA: He says no. He says as long as I'm trying to deal with it, he can wait and that my health is more important. But he is also a 21-year-old guy.

### Can You Describe a Recent and Typical Sexual Interaction?

Some clients with pelvic/sexual pain disorders may be engaging in very little or no sexual activity, while others do not have as many limitations. It is extremely helpful to ask the client to think about a recent sexual experience and describe it step by step like watching a video (Kaplan, 1995, p. 96). Make sure to ask how the client felt during the interaction and how she experienced the partner. The picture painted by the client can often reveal self-sabotage. For instance, one client described wanting to "get it over with" due to sex being painful, but in doing so, she avoided foreplay and was engaging in sex when her body was not physically ready, ensuring that she would have a painful sexual encounter.

For clients with a partner, this question can also help you to determine the partner's awareness of or reaction to the pelvic/sexual pain. Some partners misinterpret consequences from pelvic/sexual pain disorders. For example, some partners personalize the client's avoiding sexual contact or not enjoying sex. It is common to hear a partner's reactions described as sadness, hopelessness, disappointment, and even anger. If a client's partner is responding with anger, it is important to assess how the anger is being expressed and if the client is safe. If a partner is expressing anger, the client with pelvic/sexual pain might be experiencing even more pressure to perform, which in turn could make symptoms worse. I have unfortunately seen many cases when a woman with pelvic/sexual pain is complying with the sexual demands of the partner but is not actually wanting to engage in these sexual interactions. These types of interactions could be considered unwanted sexual experiences and can bring up similar occurrences from the past. Noemi's response was telling about the dynamic she and her husband were stuck in:

THERAPIST: Can you tell me about a recent sexual experience you had? Break it down for me as if I were watching it on a video.

NOEMI: Okay. . . . Last week, for instance, my husband Nick starts trying to cuddle me in bed, and I know that's his way of trying to initiate sex. He's not normally cuddly unless he wants to have sex. And I just like, physically pushed him away – like gently moved his arms away and told him I wasn't in the mood. Then he started pouting, which made me feel like total shit. He gets into such a bad mood if we don't do something sexual after about a week. It's like clockwork. So, then I just rallied, and you know, at least took care of him.

THERAPIST: Okay. What does it mean to "rally?" Walk me through that.

NOEMI: I just tell myself I need to do something for the sake of my marriage. I just gave him a hand job.

THERAPIST: Okay. Was there pleasure involved in that?

NOEMI: Maybe for him [chuckles]! He obviously was enjoying it and rubbing me and touching me over my clothes. But it just doesn't do anything for me right now. I was bored and tired and honestly just wanted to go to bed.

THERAPIST: What about afterwards?

NOEMI: He does always ask to do something for me. Always. I will give him credit for that. But I just don't want to right now. Sex just sort of feels like one more thing I have to do, not want to do. And now that it's painful, I really don't have the motivation to make it happen.

THERAPIST: How do you both feel usually after an interaction like that?

NOEMI: I feel momentary relief because at least the pressure is off. But I know it will build up again, and we really need to have sex again. That pressure is sort of always there right now. For him . . . I think he initially feels happy. He gets upset that I won't let him pleasure me in any way right now — I do think it makes him feel guilty.

### Can You Experience Pleasure During Sexual Activity? If So, How?

Some women with pelvic/sexual pain disorders have very pleasurable and fulfilling sex lives. These women usually incorporate more outercourse activities or have learned which penetrative sex positions are okay to engage in given their symptoms. Women who have been able to maintain a positive relationship with sex despite their pelvic/sexual pain disorders are less likely to have catastrophic thoughts about the impact of the disorders on their sexuality. On the other hand, women who report not being able to experience sexual pleasure may place sole blame on their pelvic/sexual pain disorder and believe they are sentenced to a life without sexual enjoyment. Many single women with pelvic/sexual pain disorders believe they will be unable to find a partner who is "willing to put up with this." Others report feeling like failures as women for being unable to engage in sexual activity with a partner or have children.

THERAPIST: You've told me that you and Nick are not having sex right now. What about outercourse? General affection?

NOEMI: At first, I was trying to occasionally just do something for him, but that has really dropped off, to be honest. Like I said, I do try and rally sometimes and do something for him once he gets moody. Right now, though, I don't even want him to touch me.

THERAPIST: Is there any type of touch that feels pleasurable right now?

NOEMI: This sounds so bad . . . but right now, no. I don't know if it's because I feel "touched out" or it's because of the trauma or both, but I don't even want a hug. I used to love to cuddle, but now I think I avoid that, too, because I don't want him to think it might lead to sex.

### What About the Emotional Connection With Your Partner? Or the Emotional Intimacy in the Relationship?

THERAPIST: You've told me that you've been unable to have penetrative sex or engage in outercourse since the accident. What about the emotional connection with your husband? Have you two been able to maintain this?

REBECCA: I don't know. Things are so different now. [crying]. Jacob always worked a lot, and I always kept myself busy with the kids and then later with my own job. We were both very independent people. And I think over our relationship, it's our traveling and little adventures together that has made our emotional intimacy so strong. But now I can't do any of that.

THERAPIST: Okay. Do you two share any enjoyable activities together now?

REBECCA: Not really. We try to have lunch together, visit the kids together. Sometimes we do a puzzle or watch a show . . . but that's so boring. . . . Jacob has basically just been my caretaker since the accident. I think that's really unattractive to both of us even though he denies it. I just feel like a burden to him.

THERAPIST: Role changes, especially unwanted and unexpected ones can be really hard to adjust to in a relationship.

REBECCA: I hate it. I know I lash out sometimes at him because of it.

### What Events in Your Life Have you Considered to be of Significant Impact?

These events could be either positive or negative events. Not specifying allows the client space to tell their own story. Clients may talk about unwanted sexual experiences when asked this question, while others may focus on family events like a move out of state or their parent's divorce. For women with pelvic/sexual pain disorders, the onset of symptoms and unfolding consequences may be discussed. Events clients consider to be of significant impact likely shaped the lens from which they see the world, including how they experience their pelvic/sexual pain disorder.

THERAPIST: What have been the most significant events in your life?

PAULA: Luckily, up until recently, I guess I've had a boring life, which is a good thing. Significant events . . . probably my grandmother dying when I was in seventh grade. I was very close with her, and she watched us a lot when we were kids. We moved for my dad's job when I was really young, but I don't even remember that. Obviously, my first relationship has been a big negative event and impacted me . . . and my entire family.

THERAPIST: Absolutely. What about any positive events? Or things that have been really meaningful or important?

PAULA: Playing soccer was a huge and happy part of my childhood. I was on some travel teams, and that was always fun. I was always close with my family, too. Yearly we always took a fun family vacation away somewhere.

### Who Are You Closest With in Your Life? Who Makes Up Your Support System?

Determining the client's current social supports has implications for the types of interventions might suggest and even the course of treatment. Without enough social support for instance, it may be difficult for a client with young children to attend pelvic floor physical therapy. In addition, interventions like eye movement desensitization and reprocessing therapy should only be conducted if the client has an adequate support system. If a client lacks enough social support, it is important to note whether this is a lifelong problem and something that existed prior to their pelvic/sexual pain disorder or whether it seems to be a negative consequence of having a pelvic/sexual pain disorder. Many women with chronic pelvic/sexual pain conditions can become socially isolated from others due to the impact on daily functioning and feeling different than others.

THERAPIST: Who makes up your support system?

REBECCA: Obviously, my husband Jacob, who is pretty much my at-home nurse and chauffer. I'm closer with my daughter than my son. I just don't get to see my son and the grandkids that much because having to be in a car is so difficult for me. And I don't know if he's just busy with his own life, you know, two kids under age five, or if he doesn't like seeing me like this? I just get the sense he doesn't want to be around me as much.

THERAPIST: What about your friends? It seems like you and Jacob have always had a lot of friends even though you have moved so many different places.

REBECCA: I've lost most of my friends. Some I still talk on the phone with. Vera, my best friend from growing up, we met at camp, and Lucy, my best friend from when we lived in England, we still talk a lot. But I don't even have anything to share other than depressing stagnant medical news [tearful]. I'm such a drag.

THERAPIST: Since the accident, it seems your social support has changed drastically.

REBECCA: Yes, because I can't do anything! I actually used to do things with my girlfriends. And I used to have friends at work, and I used to be on a volunteer committee at the synagogue. Now I'm just at home all day.

## Assessment as an Unfolding Process

The initial sessions with the client are considered a formal assessment, but assessment will continue over time. It is normal for clients not to disclose everything upfront, especially when it comes to trauma. In addition, many clients with pelvic/sexual pain disorders are hesitant about sharing just how much their symptoms have impacted them, especially if they have been dismissed by others or have been made to feel that they are being "dramatic." Other clients need to establish a connection and know the therapist is a safe person before sharing more details about their traumatic experiences.

In other cases, the client is still trying to put the pieces together and may not have the words yet to capture their experience. The client may need the assessment phase of treatment to better understand their story. The assessment may also bring up events or aspects of their trauma or pelvic/sexual pain disorder that they have not thought about in a particular way before. For instance, some clients have never been asked how their pelvic/sexual pain disorder may have impacted their careers before. Once they start to consider the answer to this question, they may find there has been a bigger impact than they have realized. The client may continue to process these events and aspects as the therapy continues. A thorough assessment is imperative in establishing appropriate treatment goals, which will be discussed in the next chapter.

## Important Takeaways

- Assessment is imperative because it will help to determine the therapy goals and the most immediate needs in treatment.
- Assessment is both a formal and informal process that unfolds over time. Assessment includes the interweave of culturally competent knowledge, awareness, and skills.
- Clinicians should create a genogram and obtain an extensive history that addresses medical/physiological factors, psychological factors, relational factors, and sociocultural factors.
- Assessment questions should consider the history of the pelvic/sexual pain disorder, the current symptoms, and the impact of the client's pelvic/sexual pain disorder on education/career, financial stability, relationships, and general quality of life.

## References

Berman, E., & Hof, L. (1987). The sexual genogram: Assessing family-of-origin factors in the treatment of sexual dysfunctions. In G. Weeks & L. Hof (Eds.), *Integrating sex and marital therapy: A clinical guide* (pp. 37–56). Brunner/Mazel.

Bowen, M. (1978). *Family therapy in clinical practice.* Aronson.

Bowen, M. (1980). Key to the use of the genogram. In E. A. Carter & M. McGoldrick (Eds.), *The family life cycle: A framework for family therapy* (p. XXIII). Gardner Press.

DeMaria, R., Weeks, G., & Hof, L. (1999). *Focused genograms: Intergenerational assessment of individuals, couples, and families.* Brunner/Mazel.

DeMaria, R., Weeks, G., & Twist, M. (2017). *Focused genograms: Intergenerational assessment of individuals, couples, and families* (2nd ed.). Routledge.

Ho, D. Y. F. (1995). Internalized culture, culturocentrism, and transcendence. *The Counseling Psychologist, 23*(1), 4–24.

Kaplan, H. S. (1983). *The evaluation of sexual disorders: Psychological and medical aspects.* Brunner/Mazel.

Kaplan, H. S. (1995). *The sexual desire disorders: Dysfunction regulation of sexual motivation.* Brunner/Mazel.

Lee, C. (2013). The cross-cultural encounter: Meeting the challenge of culturally competent counseling In C. Lee (Ed.), *Multicultural issues in counseling: New approaches to diversity* (4th ed., pp. 13–19). American Counseling Association.

Lee, C., & Park, D. (2013). A conceptual framework for counseling across cultures. In C. Lee & D. Park (Eds.), *Multicultural issues in counseling: New approaches to diversity* (4th ed., pp. 3–12). American Counseling Association.

Lee, E. (2015). How to critically use globally discerned case studies in local contexts. In R. Moodley, M. Lengyell, R. Wu, & U. Gielen (Eds.), *International counseling: Case Studies handbook* (pp. 3–11). American Counseling Association.

McGoldrick, M., Gerson, R., & Petry, S. (2008). *Genograms: Assessment and intervention* (3rd ed.). W. W. Norton & Company.

Moodley, R., Lengyell, M., Wu, R., & Gielen, U. (Eds.). (2015). *International counseling: Case studies handbook*. American Counseling Association.

Sue, D. W., & Sue, D. (2015). *Counseling the culturally diverse: Theory and practice* (7th ed.). John Wiley & Sons, Inc.

# 6

---

# ESTABLISHING APPROPRIATE
# TREATMENT GOALS

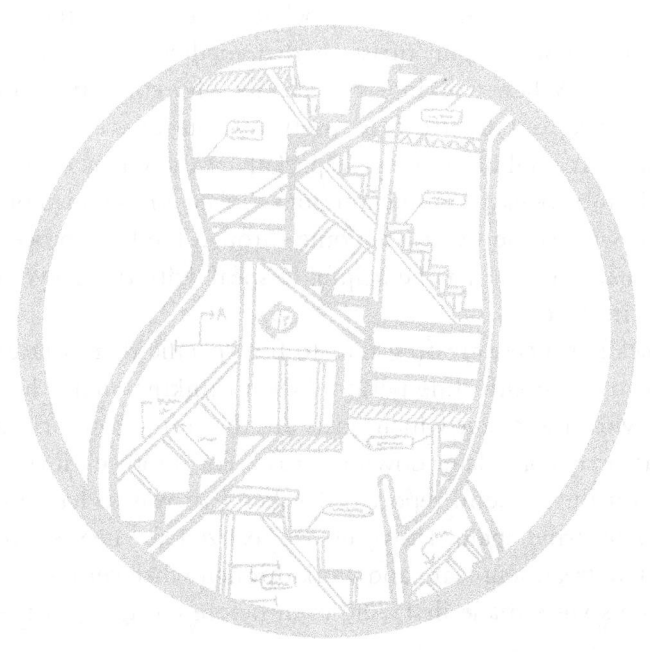

DOI: 10.4324/9781003168232-6

## Guidelines for Goal Setting

Some clients may state their goals for therapy during the first session, while others struggle with identifying what a therapeutic goal may look like. Regardless of the client's confidence in determining their goals, the assessment will guide the establishment of goals and help you to identify an order of the goals with the client. All goals should be created jointly with the client and may change as you gather more information from the client. Clients with traumatic pasts may need time to develop enough rapport with the therapist to disclose their traumas. If the consequences of these traumatic events are still impacting the client's life, then relevant goals should be created with the client to address this.

In addition, when establishing goals with clients, look for opportunities to engage with other healthcare providers involved in the client's care. Many research studies have supported the need for a multimodal approach and have demonstrated the effectiveness of collaborative care when treating vaginismus and pelvic/sexual pain (Reissing et al., 2003; Brotto et al., 2015; Bergeron et al., 2015). When working with women who have pelvic/sexual pain, it may be useful to coordinate care with a primary care provider, OB/GYN, pelvic floor physical therapist, dietitian, psychiatrist, acupuncturist, herbal medicine specialist, massage therapist, etc. When working with clients who come from more conservative backgrounds, it can be useful to consult with their religious leader such as a rabbi or priest, especially if the client believes any of the medical or behavioral interventions violate a religious norm. When working with women who are going through the legal process regarding a sexual crime, it may be helpful to speak with the lawyer or victim advocate in the case.

I typically suggest creating four to five specific therapeutic goals for a three- to six-month time period. When thinking about the timeline, identify with the client which goals are the immediate priority versus goals that may come later down the road. For instance, during our first session together, Noemi reported that her goal was to have intercourse with her husband again. However, we realized she needed to establish an effective treatment team and work through whatever medical recommendations were made first. And even before engaging in the medical treatment, we realized she needed to process the traumatic memories that had been resurfacing since having pelvic/sexual pain. The ordering of the goals must make sense to, and resonate with the client; otherwise, compliance will prove difficult.

## Broadening the Goals

To prevent clients from feeling even more stuck than they typically do, make sure to broaden the goals (Figure 6.1). For example, Siobhan identified wanting to be able to assert her physical boundaries with her husband while working through the steps of her exposure therapy ladder to treat her vaginismus. When she identified this goal, we explored what it was like for her to assert boundaries in other areas of her life outside of the intimate relationship with her husband. Through this discussion, she acknowledged always struggling with setting boundaries. Siobhan stated that since childhood, she struggled with setting boundaries with her family, which now as an adult continued, creating lots of conflict in her marriage due to her sister's taking advantage of her offers of help with childcare. This directly impacted her work related to trying to resolve her vaginismus, as she found herself time poor due to babysitting for her sister. Siobhan also realized she was allowing a coworker to take credit for her own work and that she needed to set firm boundaries with this person. Broadening this goal helped her to realize that this was not just a sex-specific issue.

Movement with a goal, either related to pelvic/sexual pain or in another area of life, will help a client to build skills and confidence. Any movement is good for therapeutic progress, even if the movement is not directly related to treating pelvic/sexual pain. For each goal, I find it useful to identify if the goal is specific to pelvic/sexual pain or if it can be broadened to any other areas of the client's life and vice versa. When attempting to broaden the goals, look for how the presenting issues might apply to the client's other relationships, including friendships, family relationships, relationships with coworkers, etc., or how the presenting problems might impact school or work performance or the ability to engage in hobbies or other enjoyable activities.

| Pelvic Pain/Sexual Goal | Related Goal |
| --- | --- |
| Be more assertive with doctor & have more control over my treatment | Be more assertive and direct with supervisor at work |
| Identify activities I find sexually pleasurable outside of penetrative sex | Identify activities or hobbies that give me joy |
| Be more direct about what I need from my partner in the moment | Be more direct with family when they set unrealistic expectations of me |
| Reduce anticipatory anxiety about sex | Reduce anxiety about presentations for work |

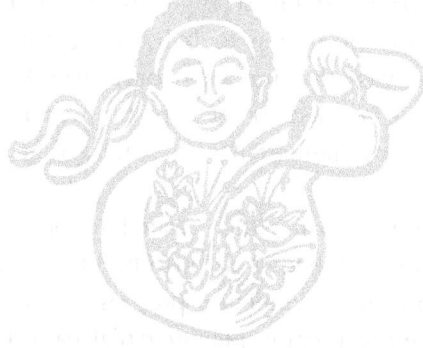

*Movement in either category will build skills and confidence... making client more likely to be able to make movement in the other category*

A goal that may seem unrelated to pelvic/sexual pain on the surface, like, for instance, better managing obsessive-compulsive disorder (OCD) symptoms, does usually have some component that impacts the pelvic/ sexual pain disorder. Many of my clients find that the OCD compulsions interfere with the treatment of their pelvic/sexual pain disorder. One client with OCD aimed to find more effective strategies for managing the symptoms due to the negative impact it was having on her work productivity. However, upon further exploration, we realized her OCD was also interfering with her ability to engage in the work needed to treat her pelvic floor dysfunction. She had to clean the dilators and wash her hands so many times that the time she set aside to do these exercises would be over before she could even begin her dilator exercises. With this insight, the client was able to see how better management of her OCD overall would also positively impact her treatment of her pelvic/sexual pain.

## Common Goals

### *Establish an Effective Treatment Team*

Very rarely will clients come to you already having an effective treatment team. I often see clients who have one provider they feel supported by but lack a diagnosis or long-term treatment plan. Others may have already run through a series of healthcare providers yet still lack an understanding of how to best manage their condition. Establishing an effective treatment team is imperative for clients regardless of their pelvic/sexual pain diagnosis. This goal requires counselors to be connected to the healthcare providers in their local community that treat people with these disorders. If you are struggling with finding pelvic/sexual pain specialists in your area, try connecting with pelvic floor physical therapists in the region. They are usually well connected to physicians and other healthcare providers in their geographical area who treat pelvic/sexual pain.

In creating a treatment team, you should first obtain a release of information from the client to speak with the other healthcare providers already involved in their care. Speaking with these providers may provide you with information about the client that you would not have known otherwise and can help you to assess for existing gaps in the treatment team. Some clients may only need a treatment team of two of three providers, including the counselor. Others may have a far more extensive team consisting of a whole range of health-care professionals. Common healthcare professionals counselors may find themselves collaborating with when treating clients with pelvic/sexual pain include OB/GYN specialists, primary care doctors, uro-gynecologists, pelvic floor physical therapists, acupuncturists, dietitians, Reiki or alternative medicine specialists, massage therapists, and psychiatrists.

Based on the presentation of symptoms, the client's history with other healthcare providers, and their current emotional state, you will want to make a referral that is an appropriate fit for the client. For instance, one client I worked with felt bullied by past healthcare providers and was very nervous about trying to address her vulvodynia with a physician. She also had a negative experience before with receiving a nerve block. After discussing her options of vulvodynia specialists in our area, the client decided to make an appointment with the doctor who was known for having a slower approach to treating patients with vulvodynia (relying more on topical creams, physical therapy, and dilator therapy) versus the more well-known doctor who relied more on injections.

Sometimes clients want the pelvic/sexual pain issue to be the immediate and sometimes only focus in therapy despite being in poor mental health or overwhelmed by trauma symptoms. For clients in this state, I encourage first trying to get their mental health in a better place so that they can engage in the work required to address their pelvic/sexual pain disorder. Not all clients heed this advice. It sometimes takes clients the experience of going to see a specialist, or sometimes beginning a treatment, to realize they need to slow down a bit. Noemi wanted to address her pelvic/sexual pain immediately despite experiencing significant posttraumatic stress disorder (PTSD) symptoms that were interfering with her daily functioning. After attending her first appointment with the pelvic floor physical therapist, she admitted feeling triggered and very vulnerable during the appointment. When this happens for clients, I try to positively reframe these experiences. It is often useful to say something like, "This is really good information and tells us where you are. It seems like we need to address your trauma symptoms before you're able to do pelvic floor physical therapy." I also try to tell clients that it is normal and expected to change course.

### Develop Assertiveness Skills

Many women with pelvic/sexual pain have spent years trying to convince healthcare providers and others in their lives that something is wrong. After years of dismissals or being told "it's all in your head," learned helplessness can set in, and women stop advocating for themselves. In addition, many women have not been socialized to be assertive but rather to be passive, accommodating, and polite. Navigating our healthcare system unfortunately requires people to be assertive, sometimes demanding, and frankly sometimes not polite.

Often women with pelvic/sexual pain need help developing assertiveness skills not only for interacting with healthcare providers but also for interacting with a partner, family, coworkers, and friends. This goal may be further complicated for women with sexual trauma who responded using the "fawn" or "freeze" response. These clients may default to behaving in an accommodating or passive state when they feel threatened. Others shut down completely. It is important to note that these responses are often activated regardless of the actual threat level but are rather evoked by just feeling threatened.

### Better Manage Chronic Pain Symptoms and Consequences

The reality is that for some women with pelvic/sexual pain conditions, chronic pain and/or physical limitations are things that they will always need to contend with. The chronic pain and/or physical limitations may impact the client's sexual functioning, ability to work, ability to engage with people important in their lives, and daily functioning such as being able to run errands or exercise. Being able to effectively manage chronic pain will enable clients to engage in activities that are important to them. It is important that women feel that although their chronic pain may always be a part of their lives, it does not have to dictate their entire lives.

## *Learn Effective Coping Skills for Anxiety and/or Depression*

Women with pelvic/sexual pain disorders often suffer from anxiety and/or depression. Anxiety and depression can interfere with clients' abilities to manage their pelvic/sexual pain conditions, as well as life in general. In fact, any mental health condition, whether PTSD or OCD, will need to be well managed before a client can turn their attention to their pelvic/sexual pain condition. Often the treating counselor who the client sought out to help treat their pelvic/sexual pain will be able to treat the other presenting mental health concerns. However, we all need to understand our limits in expertise. The client may need to work with a mental health professional who specifically specializes in treating their mental health disorder before they are able to treat their pelvic/sexual pain. Counselors should make referrals to other mental health professionals, including psychiatrists for medication consults, when appropriate.

## *Process Trauma*

Clients often come to us with a history of traumatic experiences. Clients with pelvic/sexual pain might find that their condition is stirring up old traumatic memories that they believed to be resolved or at least thought that these memories were no longer impacting them. If triggered by old traumatic memories, obtaining recommended medical treatment for their pelvic/sexual pain disorder might become too difficult. Specific treatments such as internal manipulation by a pelvic floor physical therapist, using dilators, or receiving injections may trigger the traumatic memories. If the feelings become too unmanageable, clients may avoid treatment altogether, only worsening their symptoms. Clinicians need to determine what specific traumatic memories are inferring with the client's wellbeing and ability to engage in needed treatment or care.

Sexual trauma and medical trauma are two types of traumas that commonly interfere with the treatment of women with pelvic/sexual pain disorders. However, there are a whole range of traumatic experiences, including childhood neglect, abandonment as a child, and bullying as a child, that could impact a woman's ability to engage in needed care.

Generally, any trauma that created a negative body image, caused distrust of those in authority positions, created a need to always be in control, or contributed to dissociation could interfere with treatment.

## Increase Sexual Desire

Many women with pelvic/sexual pain report having low sexual desire, and they often fail to recognize how having pain with sex contributes to their low sexual desire. Consciously or unconsciously, some women with pelvic/sexual pain may avoid sexual contact to avoid triggering their symptoms. They may label this avoidance as "low sexual desire." Psychoeducation is often needed to explain how low sexual desire may be at least partly due to the pelvic/sexual pain condition. I commonly use Emily Nagoski's *Come As You Are* (2015) as a resource for women seeking help with low sexual desire. It is imperative that women understand that while men have spontaneous desire, women have receptive or responsive desire. Only when women stop comparing themselves with the male sexual response cycle can they take ownership of the factors that either increase or decrease their sexual desire.

Other factors that can contribute to low sexual desire in women should be screened for. Factors include having a negative body image, experiencing a lack of sleep, feeling emotionally disconnected from a partner, having high stress levels, feeling triggered by unresolved trauma, dealing with anxiety/depression symptoms, and being on certain medications such as selective serotonin reuptake inhibitors or oral birth control pills. In addition, women who are breastfeeding or those who have young children may feel "touched out" and may find themselves avoiding physical intimacy from their partners. Some women with "low sexual desire" are not enjoying the type of sex they are having with their partner or are not experiencing pleasure during sex, making motivation to engage sexually quite low. For women with partners who have a much higher sexual drive and whose partners are always initiating, there may simply never be enough space or opportunity for their desire to emerge.

Many women will want to "cure" their low sexual desire first, or at the same time, as their pelvic/sexual pain. Until the factors contributing to low sexual desire are addressed, including having pain with sex or experiencing chronic fatigue from a pelvic/sexual pain condition like endometriosis, it is unlikely that sexual desire will increase. Until the client is no longer having pain with penetration, it may be difficult work on the goal of increasing low sexual desire. While dealing with the pelvic/sexual pain condition, some clients can work on increasing sexual desire towards outercourse activities, while others do not notice a shift in desire until their condition is much more managed and they are not having painful sex and disruptive daily symptoms. Therapists should have realistic conversations with clients about when and how the goal of increasing low sexual desire may be achieved rather than setting up women with pelvic/sexual pain for unrealistic expectations about increasing sexual desire. Working prematurely on this goal can cause further hits to women's self-esteem and sexual confidence, as lack of progress with increasing their sexual desire becomes another way they have "failed as a woman."

### Improve Emotional and Sexual Intimacy

For clients who are partnered, a common goal is to improve emotional and sexual intimacy. I often like clients to focus on this goal first before tackling the goal of "increasing sexual desire." Clients with pelvic/sexual pain disorders usually report a decrease in sexual intimacy with their partners, low sexual desire, and sometimes general relationship dissatisfaction. The partner with pelvic/sexual pain may find it hard to crave something that is painful and that may trigger a range of upsetting feelings like shame, disgust, anger, frustration, or feeling "not good enough." In addition, living with a chronic pain condition can be physically draining, making interest in sex even lower.

The partner without chronic pelvic/sexual pain may have withdrawn affection over time due to frustrations with their attempts at physical or sexual connection being rejected. Partners may question whether they are desirable or if the client with pelvic/sexual pain wants to be in the committed relationship. Sometimes a client's partner may need to be referred to their own counseling if they are struggling with feelings of rejection, frustration, sadness, anger, etc. about how the pelvic/sexual pain condition has impacted the relationship. It is also useful to refer a client's partner to counseling if the client's partner admits not agreeing to the client's pelvic/sexual pain treatment plan. It is imperative that the partner understand the course of treatment and their role in any of the treatment goals. It is also important partners understand how they can be supportive of their partner with pelvic/sexual pain.

Clients often need to foster more emotional and sexual intimacy while working towards the goal of reestablishing penetrative sex. Without doing this, many clients will find themselves eventually physical ready to have sex again but emotionally unprepared. I highly recommend "taking sex off the table" officially, even if couples are not engaging in penetrative sex. Once the pressure of penetrative sex is removed, the couple can work on pleasurable touch with the goal of slowly expanding the sexual repertoire to include more outercourse activities.

### Increase Pleasure

Clients often seek to increase pleasure with sexual activity, as having a pelvic/sexual pain disorder may have interfered with the enjoyment of sex. Clients may need help identifying what specific sensual or sexual activities are pleasurable. For clients also presenting with low sexual desire, it is often helpful to start with sensual bath or sensual massage. Both activities can be done solo or with a partner. As part of increasing pleasure, clients should work on making their living spaces more relaxing or sensual. For example, clients who are starting with a sensual bath could try adding candles, music, or scents to the experience. Once clients begin to enjoy sensual activities, they can progress to more sexual activities.

Beyond sex, however, I often find that women with pelvic/sexual pain need help increasing pleasure in terms of overall life enjoyment. As discussed earlier in this book, having a pelvic/sexual pain condition takes a negative toll on many aspects of a client's life. Clients may feel that their pelvic/sexual pain has forced them to lead a more restricted life, or as Rebecca put it, "This pain has robbed me of the joy in life." It can be rewarding and empowering for women reengage with activities they used to find enjoyable as they make progress in treatment. These activities usually need to be modified to meet their current abilities, and some clients may struggle to make this psychological adjustment.

## Foster Healthy and Effective Dating Skills

For clients who are single and want to date, identifying healthy and effective dating skills is essential. Many single women with pelvic/ sexual pain conditions report anxiety around dating, especially young women who may feel social pressure to engage in sexual activity early into dating someone. What might be an exciting sensual adventure with a new partner to a woman without pelvic/sexual pain is likely an anxiety-ridden experience predicted to end in "failure" or becomes something to "suffer through" for a woman with pelvic/sexual pain. Women with pelvic/sexual pain may need help establishing healthy boundaries in dating that will set them up for successful experiences with sexual intimacy rather than continuing to engage in a pattern of self-defeating behavior.

Many women with pelvic/sexual pain who are dating discuss their conflicting emotions about how and when to disclose their condition without even considering whether a potential partner has shown to be worthy of such a disclosure. I encourage women to go on at least three to five dates to determine if this potential partner is someone who they would like to date more seriously. If not, no disclosure is needed! If the dates do go well, it may be appropriate to disclose something about having a pelvic/sexual pain condition. However, it is always good to remind clients that disclosure happens on a spectrum. What one might disclose early in dating about their condition looks very different after dating for months and establishing more emotional intimacy.

Over the course of dating, if the couple has a strong connection, most partners are open to learning about and working around the pelvic/ sexual pain condition. If the potential partner decides to stop dating the woman after learning about her pelvic/sexual pain condition, it is help- ful to reframe this experience as "What does this tell us about him/her/ them as a person and possible partner?" It could simply mean penetrative sex is important to this person, but it could also mean that the person puts too much focus on penetrative sex. It might also mean they do not have much resiliency and are not someone who will stick around when things get hard in life, as they inevitably will.

I often hear women talk about how "unfair" it is that a person should have to be with someone with a pelvic/sexual pain condition without taking the time to evaluate what their potential partner might bring to the table – both good and bad. Other single women enter the dating scene knowing they are unable to have children due to their pelvic/sexual pain condition, believing this marks them as "damaged goods." Unfortunately, I have seen many women with pelvic/sexual pain conditions settle for partners who treat them poorly because they do not believe they will find someone better. If this is the case, clients may need help eventually getting out of these relationships, as counseling typically reveals how unhealthy the relationship is. These clients may need reassurance around the possibility of finding a healthy partner and having a healthy relationship despite having a pelvic/sexual pain disorder.

### Develop Stress Management Skills

Some clients need help with developing more effective stress management skills. Resiliency and the ability to cope with stressful situations is imperative for women with pelvic/sexual pain disorders. Women may need to learn to balance treatment for their pelvic/sexual pain conditions with the other demands of life. This becomes even more important for clients who have chronic pelvic/sexual pain conditions who will always have to manage some aspect their condition.

Many clients, if they have not already noticed the connection, discover while in counseling how their stress level impacts their pelvic/sexual pain condition. More stress generally increases the intensity or frequency of symptoms. Remember, stress is inflammatory. Once clients discover how stress specifically impacts their pelvic/sexual pain disorder, they may be more motivated to work on managing their stress. It can be important to remind clients that while they cannot control all of the factors that exacerbate their pelvic/sexual pain, stress management is one factor they can control, giving them the power to reduce their pain.

### Increase Self-Esteem

Many clients struggle with low self-esteem, but I find that women who have been ignored by others for years over health concerns have suffered a particular blow to their self-esteem. In addition, women who have had unwanted sexual experiences or have had other major betrayals (e.g., having a partner be unfaithful or being abandoned by a parent as a child) commonly need to work towards increasing self-esteem. Clients with betrayal experiences often need to learn to "trust their gut" and believe in their judgement.

Pelvic/sexual pain disorders also directly impact the way clients view themselves as women. Many clients discuss feeling "broken" or "not a woman" if they cannot have penetrative sex or have children. This "less than" feeling usually follows clients into many areas of their lives. Clients will need to know their value in various roles in life, including at work, with their family, as a partner, and as a sexual being – despite limitations caused by their pelvic/sexual pain disorder.

### Increase Flexibility and Creativity

This goal could be specifically about sex, like, for instance, needing to expand the sexual repertoire to include more non-penetrative sexual activities. It may also mean being flexible about the time of day for engaging in sexual activities, allowing women to have sex under more ideal conditions (e.g., when they are less tired or less stressed, which for many can result in a decrease of symptoms). It can also be beneficial to add toys for more variation and pleasure.

Outside of sex, increasing flexibility and creativity has implications for other areas of life. Clients may need help working around or working with the limitations of their pelvic/sexual pain condition when it comes work, family, friends, hobbies, etc. Perhaps a client can no longer go on long runs without provoking their symptoms, but they can swim or go on long walks. Other clients must adjust how they manage their work-day. Some clients may need to request a standing desk or a yoga ball seat. Others find they need to take a five-minute walk every hour or stretch for a few minutes. One of the silver linings of the pandemic for women with pelvic/sexual pain disorders is that they have made their work-from-home environments more conducive to managing their pelvic/sexual pain.

### Process Grief

Both in trauma work and when working with pelvic/sexual pain, grief over what could have been usually surfaces once clients are no longer in crisis. When dealing with grief associated with pelvic/ sexual pain disorders, clients may need to grieve the losses associated with their conditions, as a prerequisite for working towards successful management of their symptoms. I find this to be especially true for young women whose fertility has been impacted. The ripple effects of both traumatic experiences and pelvic/sexual pain may continue to play out in the client's life, and thus the issue of grief may continue to resurface. Clients must be able to experience and move through the grief, so it does not sit in the pelvis or somewhere else in the body.

### Identify Healthy Ways to Express Anger

Some women have difficultly being with their anger because they have been socialized to believe anger is a "bad" emotion. Unfortunately, that anger goes somewhere – whether settling in the body somewhere as tension and pain or turning into feelings of depression. Clients may need assistance in accessing their anger and learning to express their anger in healthy ways. Women tend to be penalized socially for expressing anger even when it is done in appropriate and healthy ways, so there may also need to be some psychoeducation about how to cope with this.

## When to Refer Out for Couples Therapy

When clients are partnered, it is always helpful to invite the partner in a few sessions. It is important to note that these sessions are not couples therapy sessions, and the client and partner must understand this from the start. The focus of these sessions is to get the partner on board with the treatment plan and for them to understand the treatment process. Meeting a client's partner can be extremely helpful in making sure that the client and partner share common goals and have realistic expectations about treatment. Sometimes partners underestimate the amount of work involved in treating a woman with a pelvic/ sexual pain condition and the length of time needed before resuming penetrative sex. I also discuss with the partner how they can be supportive or helpful during the treatment process.

If a partner is not supportive or you have concerns about abuse, the individual work you do with the client may shift. I have unfortunately seen many cases when a client was in an abusive relationship while also suffering from a pelvic/sexual pain condition. In addition to the traditional red flags of partner abuse, a woman with pelvic/sexual pain may experience an inordinate amount of pressure to engage in sexual activity despite their pain. Abusive partners may threaten to cheat on or leave their partner who is experiencing pelvic/sexual pain. Finally, I want to mention "weaponized incompetence." This may look like the client with pelvic/sexual pain having to take on all or most of the household or childcare activities due to their partner's inability or unwillingness to help. This prevents clients from getting the medical and psychological care they need.

I refer out to couples therapy when it is clear the couple is experiencing significant distress, especially outside of the pelvic/sexual pain issue, or if the partner or client describes the relationship as being in a crisis or "at a breaking point." I highly recommend the couples therapist be a certified sex therapist who has knowledge about pelvic/sexual pain disorders. Unfortunately, without an understanding of these disorders, I have seen couples' therapists engage in blaming behavior towards the woman with the pelvic/sexual pain disorder or set up unrealistic expectations in regard to the treatment and prognosis of the condition.

## Examples of Treatment Goals

For each of the case vignettes, I included the client's initial treatment goals that were established within the first few sessions of treatment and the client's treatment goals after three to six months of counseling. I believed it important to show how the goals evolve over time, especially once initial progress is made. Descriptions in quotes are to reflect the client's language.

### Paula's Initial Treatment Goals

1. Process complicated emotions related to the "ending of my first relationship."
2. Develop effective coping skills for stress (for legal proceedings, school, and managing pelvic/sexual pain).

3.  Use cognitive behavioral therapy (CBT) skills to reduce OCD compulsions and intrusive thoughts.
4.  Communicate with others (including partner and treatment team) in an assertive manner.
5.  Establish a treatment team and determine next steps for medically treating the pelvic/sexual pain (psychotherapist, psychiatrist, pelvic floor physical therapist, and OB/GYN specialist).

### Paula's Later Treatment Goals

1.  Use eye movement desensitization and reprocessing (EMDR) to process traumatic memories from coercive sexual relationship.
2.  Process anger and identify healthy expressions of anger.
3.  Continue with pelvic floor physical therapy and transition to penetrative sex when emotionally and physically ready.

### Violet's Initial Treatment Goals

1.  Develop effective coping skills for anxiety symptoms.
2.  Establish an appropriate treatment team for endometriosis and chronic pelvic pain (psychotherapist, pelvic floor physical therapist, dietitian, and acupuncturist).

### Violet's Later Treatment Goals

1.  Maintain healthy lifestyle that includes approaches that help to manage endometriosis and chronic pelvic pain.
2.  Increase self-confidence and belief in decision making ability (including knowing one's body, decisions in dating, and decisions about career).

### Rebecca's Initial Treatment Goals

1.  Develop anxiety coping skills with CBT techniques.
2.  Process past traumatic memories using EMDR therapy.

### Rebecca's Later Treatment Goals

1.  Engage in pleasurable activities daily.
2.  Continue with treatment recommended by pelvic floor physical therapist.

3.   Consult with psychiatrist.
4.   Engage in shared hobbies or interests with partner.
5.   Process grief around "what could have been" if not for the accident.
6.   Begin sensate focus exercises with partner with eventual goal of expanding outercourse repertoire.

### Siobhan's Initial Treatment Goals

1.   Reduce phobic-like responses to one's body, partner's body, and sensual touch.
2.   Develop effective anxiety coping skills.
3.   Confirm (or rule out) lifelong vaginismus diagnosis and proceed with OB/GYN specialist's recommendations (pelvic floor physical therapy and dilator therapy).
4.   Identify physical affection or intimacy that is currently not triggering and begin to engage in with partner.

### Siobhan's Later Treatment Goals

1.   Use EMDR therapy to reduce anxiety and build confidence regarding dilator therapy.
2.   Establish healthy boundaries with others (specifically with sister and other family members, coworkers, and healthcare providers).
3.   Learn skills for assertive communication (to use with partner, treatment team, family, coworkers).
4.   Continue to expand sensual and sexual activities that are enjoyable to share with partner, with the ultimate goal of adding penetrative sex (when physically and emotionally ready).

### Noemi's Initial Treatment Goals

1.   Develop coping skills for PTSD symptoms.
2.   Process traumatic experiences using EMDR therapy.
3.   Increase non-demand touch with partner.
4.   Reconnect with partner by implementing "date night."

### Noemi's Later Treatment Goals

1.   Process feelings of grief and anger.
2.   Continue expanding on sexual intimacy in preparation for penetrative sex.

3. Identify strategies to increase sexual desire.
4. "Reclaim" body.

## Important Takeaways

- Treatment goals are always created collaboratively with the client and will change as treatment progresses. Four to five treatment goals for a three- to six-month time period are recommended.
- Communication with others involved in the client's healthcare is needed for effective treatment because a multimodal approach is most effective for treatment complex sexual issues like pelvic/sexual pain.
- Broaden the treatment goals to demonstrate how pelvic/sexual pain–related goals are related to other areas of the client's life and vice versa. This will help clients to stay engaged in the treatment process and reduce feelings of being stuck.
- A partner may attend a few sessions to better understand the treatment process, establish realistic expectations, and learn how they can be supportive of the partner in treatment. Clinicians may need to refer the client and her partner to couples therapy if the couple appears to be experiencing high levels of distress or is in crisis.

## References

Bergeron, S., Corsini-Munt, S., Aerts, L., Rancourt, K., & Rosen, N. O. (2015). Female sexual pain disorders: A review of the literature on etiology and treatment. *Current Sexual Health Reports, 7*, 159–169.

Brotto, L. A., Young, P., Smith, K. B., & Sadownik, L. A. (2015). Impact of a multidisciplinary vulvodynia program on sexual functioning and dyspareunia. *The Journal of Sexual Medicine, 12*, 238–247.

Nagoski, E. (2015). *Come as you are*. Simon & Schuster.

Reissing, E. D., Binik, Y. M., Khalif, S., Cohen, D., & Amsel, R. (2003). Etiological correlates of vaginismus: Sexual and physical abuse, sexual knowledge, sexual self-schema, and relationship adjustment. *Journal of Sex & Marital Therapy, 29*(1), 47–59. doi:10.1080/713847095

# 7

# TREATMENT TECHNIQUES

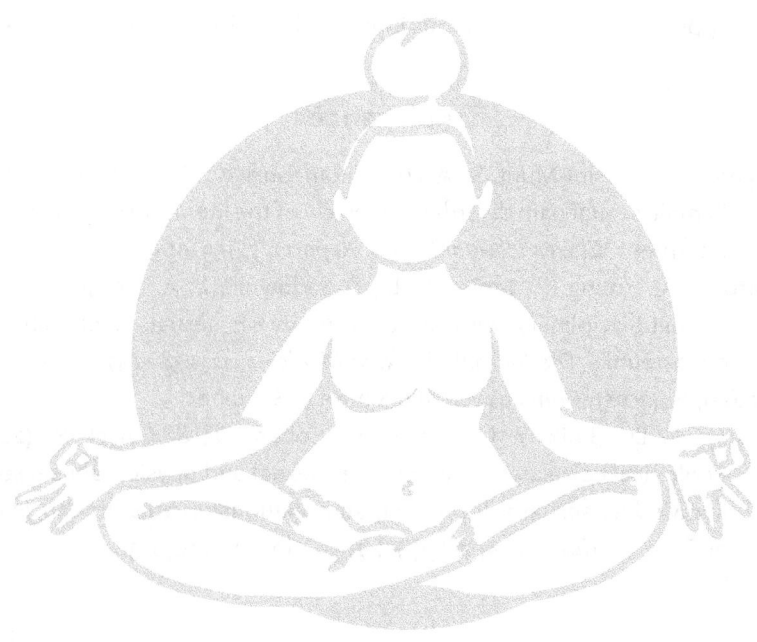

DOI: 10.4324/9781003168232-7

## A Multidisciplinary Treatment Approach

This chapter reviews evidence-based treatment techniques for treating pelvic/sexual pain and sexual trauma including graduated exposure therapy, psychoeducation, cognitive behavioral therapy, eye movement desensitization and reprocessing (EMDR) therapy, mindfulness techniques, and behavioral sex therapy interventions. While this is not an exhaustive review of treatment techniques, my hope is that clinicians learn about a range of techniques to choose from. To note, a multidisciplinary approach is recommended for complex sexual issues, such as pelvic/sexual pain and trauma-related disorders (Brotto et al., 2015; Bergeron et al., 2015).

The task of successfully implementing this type of approach, especially for mental health professionals working with women of lower socioeconomic status in a fragmented healthcare system, is daunting but possible. In my experience, several keys to a successful multidisciplinary approach involve (1) applying a wide range of evidence-based treatments to the presenting problems; (2) using culturally competent treatment strategies that address the role of gender, race, class, disability status, sexual orientation, religion, etc.; and (3) being comfortable with multiple treatment modalities (individual, couples, and group therapy) as a way to address the dyadic contributors to pelvic/sexual pain.

## Establishing an Effective Treatment Team

Every client with pelvic/sexual pain will need an effective treatment team. The task of establishing an effective treatment team can require effort on the psychotherapist's part. A multidisciplinary treatment approach requires the mental health professional to find and connect with other healthcare providers and familiarize themselves with local resources, including those that offer services on a sliding scale. Ideal professionals to collaborate with should demonstrate flexibility in modifying and scaffolding treatment to match the client's evolving needs. Collaboration with other providers involved in the client's care is crucial, as each provider will likely see some aspect of the client's presentation that the other is not able to.

A typical treatment team for a woman with a pelvic/sexual pain disorder usually includes an (1) OB/GYN who specifically treats client's sexual/pelvic pain condition, (2) a pelvic floor physical therapist, and (3) a psychotherapist who specializes in sexual/pelvic pain. The following professionals may be needed for additional support or management of factors contributing to the pelvic/sexual pain disorder:(1) primary care physician, (2) urogynecologist, (3) psychiatrist, (4) dermatologist or vulvar skin specialist, (5) rheumatologist, (6) acupuncturist, (7) registered dietitian, (8) massage therapist, (9) reiki or qigong provider, (10) herbal medicine specialist, or (11) a religious or spiritual advisor.

For psychotherapists who are struggling to find healthcare providers in their community who specialize in treating women with sexual/pelvic pain disorders, I recommend checking out the following organizations that have directories for professionals who are part of their organizations: (1) International Society for Pelvic Pain (ISPP); (2) International Society for the Study of Women's Sexual Health (ISSWSH); (3) American Association of Sex Educators, Counselors and Therapists (AASECT); (4) Herman & Wallace Pelvic Rehabilitation Institute; 5) The Interstitial Cystitis Association; (5) Endometriosis Foundation of America; and (6) National Vulvodynia Association.

Creating an appropriate treatment team is a critical part of early treatment with any client struggling with a pelvic/sexual pain disorder. As previously discussed, many women spend years visiting specialists yet lack a diagnosis or treatment strategy for their pelvic/sexual pain. Many feel dismissed and unseen by the medical community at best and traumatized by the medical community at worst. On the surface, the task of establishing an effective treatment team may seem purely logistical. Which pelvic floor physical therapist is most convenient in terms of location and hours for the client? Is this sliding scale acupuncturist familiar with the client's specific pelvic/sexual pain disorder? Does this medical specialist accept the client's insurance? These are all relevant and important logistical questions when establishing an effective treatment team.

These basic logistical questions may present as very triggering and overwhelming for women with negative experiences with the medical community. Many women I have worked with report experiencing very high levels of anxiety when interacting with medical providers or their insurance companies. After finally finding a pelvic floor physical therapist who accepted Violet's health insurance, her employer changed their HMO a few months into treatment. Luckily, the new plan still covered Violet's care. However, before this could be confirmed, the news of changing health insurance put Violet into a tailspin. She cried hysterically in session about finally finding a provider who was helpful and anticipated its being ripped away from her. It also triggered her trauma around financial insecurity, something that followed her into adulthood due to student loan debt.

Noemi also struggled with navigating the process of setting up care with providers. Still trapped in a trauma state from her traumatic birth experience and angered by the circus of fighting her insurance company for coverage of an event that nearly killed her, upon receiving a statement from the health insurance company, Noemi would either "push it away" by shoving the unopened letters into a pile on the dining room table or nearly have a panic attack thinking about having to call the insurance company again. Her approach in dealing with the insurance company mirrored how she was also approaching her trauma – to either "push it away" (essentially become numb) or panic, a common emotional fluctuation for those with posttraumatic stress disorder (PTSD).

It is in these early interactions with both healthcare providers and the insurance companies that highlight where the early therapeutic work may need to be done. In Violet's case, it revealed the feeling of helplessness from a lifetime of financial instability and her fears of having "picked the wrong career." The fear of picking the wrong career was linked to her core belief of not trusting her own judgement or experiences. For Noemi, her reactions highlighted how active her PTSD symptoms were, another indicator that her traumatic experiences should be dealt with early in treatment.

There are many opportunities within the goal of establishing an effective treatment team to address other goals the client may be working towards. For Violet, establishing her treatment team presented as an opportunity for her to practice assertiveness skills with the medical community and to take more ownership of her health by being more active in healthcare decisions. She later reflected that these interactions helped her to feel more empowered and helped her to begin to trust her judgment. In Noemi's battle with her health insurance company, she began to acknowledge the level of anger she had about both her sexual trauma and traumatic birth experience. Once she was able to confront these emotions, she was able to be calmer and more assertive with the health insurance company rather than avoiding or being flooded with emotion.

In an ideal world, we would be connected to a multitude of medical professionals who are trauma informed; have a warm bedside manner; have the time to listen to all our client's questions; and, of course, accept our clients' insurance plans. But the world is far from ideal. It is in the acknowledgement of a broken and fragmented healthcare system that as mental health professionals, we can help our clients with navigating this reality. For instance, in Noemi's case, the pelvic floor physical therapist who accepted her health insurance was not particularly a trauma-informed provider. I consulted with Noemi about allowing me to share with the pelvic floor physical therapist relevant aspects of Noemi's traumatic experiences and how treatment could proceed at a pace that felt sustainable for her. Consulting with the pelvic floor physical therapist proved extremely helpful, and although our 20-minute phone consult did not transform this provider into being trauma informed, it did make the pacing of treatment appropriate for Noemi and helped the pelvic floor physical therapist to be aware of Noemi's particular trauma triggers.

Sometimes the medical professionals who may be able to provide the best medical care for our clients may not be the most sensitive or have the best "bedside manner." In these situations, the work with our clients may be about preparing them for such a reality. Assertiveness skills, clear communication, and realistic expectation setting are imperative for such interactions with these medical professionals. One client desperately needed to see an endometriosis specialist; however, the provider covered by her health insurance was known to be a little gruff. The provider was an excellent surgeon and endometriosis specialist despite the poor bedside manner. Because I already knew this from another client's experience with this provider, I was able to prepare the client for what their appointment might look and feel like. I encouraged the client to focus on her specific medical questions and that she could process the emotional aspect of the appointment with me later. In setting realistic expectations about what interacting with this doctor might look like, the client was able to have a positive experience.

To set up clients for success in interacting with medical professionals, I encourage clients to focus on what they can control – their communication – not the doctor's. A study conducted in the United Kingdom examined communication between doctors and women with endometriosis. One important finding was that both doctors and their patients with endometriosis found a numeric rating scale inadequate in discussing endometriosis-related pain. Rather, both the doctors and women with endometriosis found talking about the quality, location, and impact of the pain on daily functioning to be more helpful (Bullo & Weckesser, 2021). In tune with these findings, I recommend that clients bring the following information in written format, no longer than one page, to an appointment to increase the chances of feeling and being heard by their healthcare provider:

1.  *Create a timeline:* Creating a timeline for of when the pain started may be difficult for some clients. Have the client reflect on when they first started noticing their symptoms. Clients should also reflect on life events that occurred a year before the onset of symptoms. Events may include the birth of a child, a miscarriage, a car accident, a fall, a new diagnosis of a medical condition or worsening of one, new medication, or even significant weight loss or weight gain. Also take note of life stressors within a year of when the pain started. Factors may include issues with mental health, the birth of a child, the death of a family member, significant relationship distress, a divorce, a move, being diagnosed with a chronic illness, or significant career stress. While all the details are not relevant to the doctor, the timeline will show the full scope of events leading up to and possibly contributing to the pain.

2.  *Use a pain scale:* A detailed pain scale will be discussed in this chapter. Having a pain scale for reference is extremely helpful for clients to be able to see how their pains changes over time. Have clients note how and when the pain changes. Clients should be able to identify their daily baseline pain versus their level of pain when experiencing a flare-up of symptoms. The pain scale can be useful in describing the fluctuations of the pain over a period of time.

3.  *Type of pain:* Clients who can describe the type of pain to a healthcare provider may increase their odds of getting to a specialist who is an appropriate fit. Have clients consider whether the pain is dull, throbbing, stabbing, sharp, mild, stinging, burning, aching, itchy,

etc. Clients should note whether the type of pain changes based on activity or time of day.

4.  *Location*: Clients should be able to specifically communicate where their pain is. Unfortunately, many women lack basic education about their genital area, and many do not know the difference between the vagina and vulva. Psychoeducation is needed before clients attend appointments with medical specialists so they can clearly communicate where they feel the pain or discomfort. Clients should also note whether the pain always stays in that location or if it moves or shifts based on certain changes. Using the pain scale to communicate the differences in severity of pain, especially if there are multiple areas of pain, can be extremely helpful. Guide clients on using clear and specific language. For instance, "It hurts everywhere down there" is not as helpful as "It hurts around my vaginal opening" or "I have vulvar pain."

5.  *When*: Healthcare providers need to know when the pain occurs. Is the pain only provoked by certain activities, like penetrative sex for instance? Or perhaps only during certain times of the client's cycle? Again, helping clients to be specific is helpful in communicating with their healthcare provider. For instance, "It hurts all of the time" is not as helpful as "The pain is always there, but it is worse after sex."

## Graduated Exposure Therapy

Any effective treatment plan will first meet the client where they are. Creating a graduated exposure therapy ladder with the client early in treatment provides more information as to the specific steps required to meet the client's goals. It serves to identify both the starting point and the end goals, which are different for each client (Figure 7.1). The first step, or bottom step, indicates the work that must be done first before progressing to the second step. The final step includes the long-term or ultimate goals such as achieving penetrative sex or being able to tolerate a pelvic exam.

For patients like Siobhan with lifelong vaginismus, for instance, the first step often involves basic sex education and exposure around one's own genitalia. Until a client learns basic anatomy and can be comfortable

# Treatment Techniques:
## Graduated Exposure Therapy

*You must meet
the client
where they are.*

Confident
sexually, broad
sexual menu

"Parking the car"

Insertion of dilator #4

Insertion of dilator #2,
Once comfortable, move to dilator #3

Insertion of dilator #1, range of anxiety coping skills,
processing trauma or abuse, effective communication
skills, sexual pleasure

Psychoeducation about body, sex and sexual desire, images > own
self in mirror, positive view of genetalia, basic anxiety coping
skills, assertiveness skills, holding vaginal dilator, etc.

touching and exploring, they will not be able to insert a dilator. For lifelong vaginismus cases, the beginning step could take months and involves its own series of exposure steps. Because lifelong vaginismus cases present like a phobia, these clients typically have very strong aversions and negative feelings about looking at or touching themselves. For Siobhan, we first spent time reviewing basic human anatomy and sexual education. Siobhan reported being comfortable looking at drawings of human anatomy, but the thought of looking at medical photos made her "extremely anxious and honestly repulsed." With the help of EMDR, Siobhan was able to reduce her phobic anxiety response and tolerate looking at medical images, which prepared her for her second step on her graduated exposure therapy ladder – self-exploration.

Violet, on the other hand, despite having chronic pelvic/sexual pain, was comfortable with her body and had pleasurable experiences with outercourse. Therefore, her first step was reducing her overall anxiety symptoms, followed by starting pelvic floor physical therapy. Despite having experienced a sexual assault in the past, this experience did not become a barrier to pelvic/sexual pain treatment, although it was addressed in therapy. Some women with pelvic/sexual pain may enter psychotherapy knowing they want to, and need to, address a past traumatic event. Other women may believe they have addressed their trauma in the past and are surprised to find how triggered and present the traumatic event feels since experiencing pelvic/sexual pain. Such was the case for Noemi, whose past sexual assault in the workplace came roaring back into the forefront of her memory after experiencing a traumatic birth and pelvic/sexual pain.

Traumatic events, including sexual trauma, medical trauma, and childhood abuse and neglect, typically need to be processed early in treatment. Without processing the traumatic event, women may find themselves unable to cope with the medical treatment of pelvic/sexual pain, which can often be invasive and painful. Noemi felt pressure to resume penetrative sex quickly due to marital distress and wanted to start pelvic floor physical therapy immediately despite my recommendations to first deal with the multiple traumatic events she found herself struggling with. However, after her first session with the pelvic floor physical therapist, which did involve an internal exam, she found herself very overwhelmed and agreed to first focus on the trauma. Sometimes clients need to have these experiences to reprioritize the immediate treatment goals, which will impact the exposure therapy ladder.

The exposure therapy ladder serves as an excellent way for clients to keep track of their progress. As is typical, many clients want to see immediate, and sometimes unrealistic, progress, especially those with pelvic/sexual pain. Being able to refer to the exposure therapy ladder and revisit the steps already completed can help clients to feel proud of and motivated by their successes in treatment thus far. If a client is finding their current treatment step too anxiety provoking (I recommend anxiety be no higher than a 4 of 10; see Figure 7.2 for additional details), then a "bridge step" is warranted. A bridge step is an additional step that bridges or goes in between two steps when a client reports that their anxiety is too high to complete the next step on the exposure therapy ladder.

For example, after engaging in self-exploration, Siobhan's next treatment step was to purchase a dilator set and get used to being around them. Siobhan initially experienced high anxiety even just looking at the dilators, but after "hanging out with them" while watching TV or cooking dinner and touching them to her hands and arms, she began to feel much more comfortable. The next step was for Siobhan to then "nest" the dilator at her vaginal opening but not insert it. Siobhan found herself flooded with anxiety even at the thought of touching the dilator to her vaginal opening. Because she reported this anxiety as a 7/10, we decided to create a "bridge step." I asked her to think of another step that would not push her anxiety above a 4/10. Siobhan identified touching the dilator to her inner thighs and vulva as a step forward that would not push her anxiety above a 4/10. Once Siobhan completed this bridge step, she felt more confident moving to the next step and reported that her anxiety was at a much more manageable level.

## Psychoeducation as Empowerment

As previously discussed, psychoeducation is often one of the first steps on women's graduated exposure therapy ladders. Having accurate and up-to-date knowledge can be empowering for women who have lacked such information regarding their own bodies and diagnoses for years. Common topics addressed during the psychoeducation phase

# Anxiety Scale

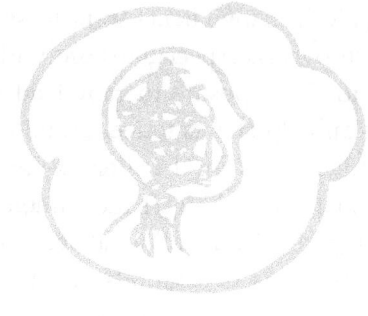

Meltdowns About
Wanting to Leave
Profession

Conflict w
Bio Dad's Family

Endometriosis
Surgery & Diagnosis

Grad School
Comp Exams

Starting
Pelvic Foor
Physical Therapy

Move to
New City

Ordering
Dilators

Traffic jam,
late to work

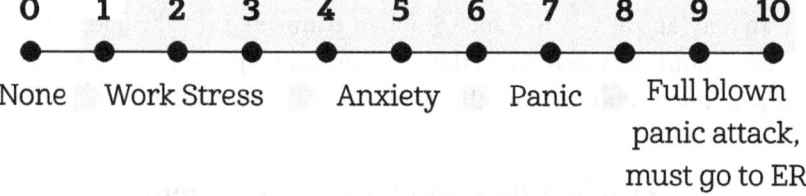

| 0 | 1 | 2 | 3 | 4 | 5 | 6 | 7 | 8 | 9 | 10 |

None    Work Stress        Anxiety        Panic        Full blown
panic attack,
must go to ER

Example: GPPPD

include human anatomy, the sexual response cycle, and identifying both medical and psychological factors contributing to pelvic/sexual pain. Time may need to be spent on challenging or dispelling sexual myths or stories clients may be telling themselves about their bodies or sexual functioning. Additionally, it is important to share the data showing that pelvic/sexual pain conditions and other related sexual concerns are very common. This can not only reduce isolation but also help clients to realize many of these common chronic issues can be managed and do not have to prevent them from living fulfilling lives.

Prior to the COVID-19 pandemic, I had a model of a woman's pelvis, including the musculoskeletal components. Together with the client, we examined the model, took the model apart, and identified the different anatomy. The pelvis model served as useful when explaining to clients the importance of pelvic floor physical therapy and dilator therapy. It also demystified the often anxiety ridden question of "Where does the dilator and/or the physical therapist's finger go?" As clients progressed through their graduated exposure therapy ladder, they often requested to see the pelvis model again, especially if they were feeling stuck or anxious.

In addition to literature containing accurate medical drawings or images of human anatomy and the female pelvis model, other resources I had in my office were an OhNut (a helpful device for when clients are ready to transition to penetrative sex), a dilator kit, a small speculum, and a tiny brush and spatula used during a Pap smear. Allowing clients to interact with these physical therapy tools and medical equipment helps in exposure and reducing anxiety. Many clients appreciated being able to hold and interact with these tools in a safe non-medical setting where they could ask questions and process their emotional reactions. Adjustments have been needed given the pandemic. While not entirely the same, the therapist can first show these materials via video, and then the client can order these materials and interact with them via a video session with the therapist. Similar exposure and emotional processing can be achieved via video. It is also extremely helpful to identify the healthcare providers in your community who provide psychoeducational pelvic exams. This is a critical part of treatment but obviously needs to be done by a medical provider. The psychoeducation phase of treatment is an appropriate time for clients to start to contact relevant healthcare professionals they will need for treatment.

## Cognitive Behavioral Therapy and Mindfulness Skills

Cognitive behavioral therapy and mindfulness skills have been shown to be effective in treating women with sexual pain (Bergeron et al., 2008; Masheb et al., 2009; Brotto et al., 2015). While this chapter is not an exhaustive inventory of all the CBT or mindfulness techniques that can be used with clients who have pelvic/sexual pain, I have included the most common techniques I use with clients.

Very early in treatment, I recommend doing a pain and anxiety scale, as it serves as a tool clinicians can use throughout the entirety of treatment and is an indicator for where the client is emotionally as they start treatment. The pain and anxiety scales are two separate scales that are used in conjunction with each other (see Figures 7.2 and 7.3, which feature Violet's case as the example). The scales are completed during a session with the client, and instructions are given on how to use them at home. On two blank pieces of paper, the client will draw a 0 to 10 scale on each piece of paper, one being the anxiety scale and the other being the pain scale.

I typically have clients start with the pain scale, as it is often easier to acknowledge physical pain rather than the possible role of anxiety. Zero marks no pain. A 10 indicates pain so severe you need to go to the emergency room. It is importance to use the description of "pain so bad you need to go to the emergency room" as a reference point because many women entering psychotherapy with unmanaged pelvic/sexual pain disorders might initially report their pain as a 10, yet it is not so severe they need to go to the hospital. Instruct the client to first list other physically painful experiences outside of their pelvic/sexual pain disorder. Try to have the client come up with about five to seven experiences unrelated to pelvic/sexual pain that are across the pain scale. If the client struggles to site experiences outside of pelvic/sexual pain, ask if the client has experienced any of the following and where they would rate the pain on the zero to ten scale: (1) stubbing a toe, (2) post-workout soreness, (3) a headache, (4) a migraine, (5) dental work including filling a cavity or getting braces, (6) back or neck pain, (7) a sprain, (8) joint stiffness or soreness, (9) pain related to the menstrual cycle, (10) an injury that needed stiches, (11) a broken bone, (12) a surgery, (13) pregnancy-related discomfort or pain, and (14) childbirth.

# Pain Scale

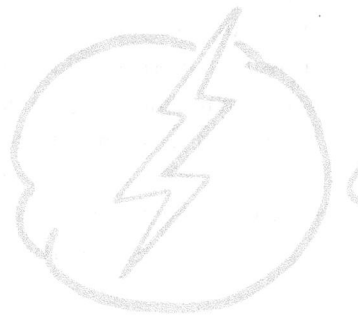

Peak of
Endometriosis
Symptoms,
Pre-Surgery

Flare-up of
Endometriosis
Symptoms
Post-Surgery

Day After
Pelvic Foor
Physical Therapy

Symptoms
Post-Surgery

Current Baseline
of Endometriosis

Headache

Inserting
Dilator #1

Soreness After
Two Mile Walk

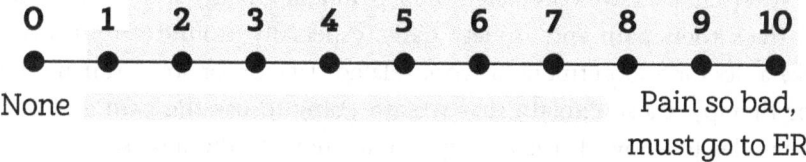

| 0 | 1 | 2 | 3 | 4 | 5 | 6 | 7 | 8 | 9 | 10 |

None                                                          Pain so bad,
must go to ER

Example: GPPPD

The next step is for the client to place experiences with their pelvic/sexual pain disorder along the pain scale, now using their unrelated painful experience as a new reference point. For some clients, their pelvic/sexual pain experiences will be their most painful experiences, but for others, once they refer to their other painful experiences, they may rate their pelvic/sexual pain experiences as moderate. Encourage clients to be very specific about the experiences. For instance, "pain with sex" is not as specific as "pain with sex in the spring of 2019 during a vulvodynia flare-up." Have clients distinguish between their daily baseline pain versus pain during a flare-up of symptoms or after a particular activity has provoked the pain.

Steps to complete the anxiety scale are similar. A 0 is no anxiety at all, while a 10 is anxiety so bad you have panic so severe you need to go to the emergency room for care. Again, have the client first note anxiety provoking experiences outside of their pelvic/sexual pain disorder across the anxiety scale. Common anxiety-provoking experiences that clients often site include (1) moving, (2) a divorce or end of a long-term relationship, (3) taking or studying for exams, (4) the death of a pet or loved one, (5) the illness of a pet or loved one, (6) a career change, (7) being stuck in traffic, (8) having a conflict with a family member or friend, (9) dealing with a difficult coworker, (10) financial insecurity or stress, and (11) stress related to the caretaker role. Next the client would add anxiety-provoking events related to their pelvic/sexual pain disorder on the scale using their events not related to pelvic/sexual pain as reference points.

After clients have completed their pain and anxiety scales, I ask them to track their pain and anxiety daily, especially around certain events like a doctor appointment, a work-related stressor, or stress during dilator therapy. I also explain that we are going to use the pain and anxiety scales to know if it is appropriate to move to the next step on their exposure therapy ladder. I instruct clients that with any step their pain should never be above a 2 of 10, and their anxiety should never be above a 4 of 10. If their anxiety or pain is above these numbers, then either more work needs to be done at the current step or a bridge step should be added. It is important to set realistic expectations. For instance, it is normal to have physical discomfort with some of these steps, and it is important to differentiate between pain and discomfort. In addition, there will likely be some level of anxiety with any step, but we do not want high levels of anxiety that could contribute to the pelvic/sexual pain by the body unconsciously clenching muscles, for example.

The pain and anxiety scales also illustrate the mind–body connection. After tracking for some time, many clients observe their pain increase as their stress and anxiety increase. Noticing this correlation helps clients realize they can at least control one factor that plays into their pelvic/ sexual pain condition – if they can work on reducing their anxiety and stress, they can reduce their pain. Tracking the pain also helps clients to identify what triggers the pain, informing them as to what activities or environmental conditions they can modify to better manage the pain.

Knowing how a certain activity might cause a flare-up of symptoms and for how long the flare-up might last can also be empowering for clients in choosing which activities are "worth it." For instance, early in treatment, Violet noted on her pain scale that long walks seemed to aggravate her pelvic floor dysfunction symptoms. Her friends invited her on a camping and hiking trip, which she reported wanting to attend but was terrified it could cause a flare-up of her symptoms. Using the data she had collected from her anxiety and pain scales in conjunction with feedback form her pelvic floor physical therapist, we discussed if there was a way she could partake in the trip. Violet decided to go but keep her hiking each day to no more than two miles on flat terrain, an amount she believed would be manageable based on her pain scale. Although she experienced a small flare-up, the experience helped Violet realize she could choose to engage in certain activities while also being mindful of not pushing her body to the point of a major flare-up.

The pain and anxiety scales are also a great way for clients to track their progress, something that can be hard for clients to see, as they can become fixated on their ultimate goals rather than seeing all of the small steps they are accomplishing to reach those ultimate goals. The scales also serve as a guide for clients, indicating when they can progress to the next step on their exposure therapy ladder. And finally, the scales can help to demystify the anxiety and pain. Once clients see the patterns in their anxiety and pain, their fear and avoidance decrease. I also encourage clients to simply notice their pain and anxiety and to view the symptoms as the body's way of communicating to them. This creates an opportunity to dialogue with the pain and anxiety rather than trying to resist or fight against it.

A mood log is another CBT technique I often use with clients struggling with pelvic/sexual pain disorders. I recommend David Burns' *The Feeling Good Handbook* (1999) as a resource for not only a mood log but also a range of CBT worksheets. After clients feel comfortable tracking their anxiety and pain, I usually have clients then start to track the thoughts that come along with their experiences of anxiety and pain. In session, I review the basic principles of CBT, including what a cognitive distortion is, the types of cognitive distortions, and the impact of our thoughts on our emotional state. Then, using the mood log, I have clients record their cognitive distortions and the types of cognitive distortions. During the following session, we review any patterns the client discovered in their thinking and how to challenge their distorted thoughts.

Just as with their experiences with pain and anxiety, it is imperative that clients also learn to notice or observe their distorted thoughts rather than react to them. Being mindful of these thoughts allows clients to slow down their emotional reactions to these thoughts. In doing so, the client can challenge the thought and shift their emotional state. Another important aspect of the mood log to the therapeutic work is that the mood log often reveals the negative core beliefs the client has about themselves. Violet's mood log, for instance, revealed her self-doubt and low self-esteem. The mood log can also show clients that the distorted thinking they face in dealing with their pelvic/sexual pain creeps into many areas of their life. Once Violet started tracking her cognitive distortions, the experience highlighted for her the extent to which self-doubt and low self-confidence plagued her life experiences in general. It also helped her to see how many of the skills she was learning to better manage her pelvic/sexual pain would help her in the other areas of her life.

One way to incorporate mindfulness skills into the CBT work with clients is to have them note the physical sensations of their anxiety and pain. If clients can be more in tune with their bodies, they can learn the early signs of their anxiety and pain increasing. For instance, Noemi noted that a 3 on her anxiety scale seemed to be correlated with a tension headache. If the anxiety or stress continued, she would later notice a flare-up in her pelvic pain. Noemi began to view the tension headache as a warning sign from her body to reduce her anxiety and stress. She learned that intervening earlier, at the sign of a tension headache, helped her to prevent a flare-up of her pelvic/sexual pain.

Teaching diaphragmatic breathing is always helpful for clients. For clients with pelvic/sexual pain, encourage them to check in with their pelvic floor physical therapist about their breathing, as breathing can impact the pelvic symptoms. Once clients learn how to engage in diaphragmatic breathing correctly, they can incorporate this breathing into stress reduction techniques and during any step on their exposure therapy ladder that causes distress. Other clients like to make note of their breathing while completing the pain and anxiety scales or a mood log, as breathing from the chest instead of the belly can be an indicator of higher stress or anxiety. Many clients will want to practice yoga to strengthen mindfulness skills. I always encourage clients to first check with their pelvic floor physical therapists before doing so, as certain poses could flare-up symptoms.

## Eye Movement Desensitization and Reprocessing Therapy

As a certified EMDR therapist, I have found EMDR extremely useful in working with clients with pelvic/sexual pain. EMDR is a structured eight-phase treatment protocol and an evidenced-based trauma treatment. In short, EMDR therapy identifies unprocessed memories containing negative beliefs, feelings, and physical sensations. Bilateral stimulation activates the brain's processing system so these memories can be processed adaptively. Clients can make meaning and gain positive insights about these memories while getting rid of the old negative scripts and stories tied to the memories. Numerous controlled studies have demonstrated EMDR's effectiveness in the treatment of trauma and has been found to be more effective than other trauma treatment methods. EMDR is effective in treating both big "T" trauma and small "t: trauma, including attachment trauma (Shapiro, 2018; Shapiro & Forrest, 2016; Shapiro, 2014; (Shapiro et al., 2007).

EMDR therapy is not appropriate for all clients. In general, clients who are a good fit for EMDR already have an established rapport with the therapist, are committed to therapy, can tolerate high levels of affect, have sufficient supports outside of therapy, and have responded well to EMDR preparatory exercises like creating a peaceful or safe place. Clients who are not a good fit for EMDR include those who cannot tolerate high levels of affect, lack supports outside of therapy, are currently engaging in substance or alcohol abuse, are currently engaging in self-harm behaviors, are in very poor health, and have or are suspected of having dissociative identity disorder. EMDR therapy cannot also be conducted with a client if the trauma is still occurring. For instance, it would not be appropriate to do EMDR therapy with a client who is being abused in her marriage. If the client can leave the marriage and establish safety, EMDR therapy could then be used to process the abuse that happened during the marriage. For clients involved in legal proceedings due to their trauma, it is imperative that they consult with their lawyers about how a resolution of their posttraumatic stress disorder (PTSD) or related symptoms due to EMDR treatment could impact their case (Parnell, 2013; Shapiro et al., 2007).

If you are not trained and certified in EMDR therapy, I highly recommend referring clients for EMDR treatment when appropriate. Resource tapping is a skill that is now used independent of EMDR therapy and can be practiced by those not trained in EMDR. Laurel Parnell's *Tapping In: A Step-by-Step Guide to Activating Your Healing Resources Through Bilateral Stimulation* (2008) is a great guide for clinicians seeking to use "resource tapping." There are several resource tapping exercises I use from this book, including creating a safe or peaceful place and creating a team of helpers that the client can channel when needed.

I recommend therapists always have clients establish a safe or peaceful place and create a team of helpers early into treatment, as I find that both are needed often as clients confront traumatic experiences and attempt to overcome their anxieties or fears. In creating the team of helpers, I recommend the client identify three for each of the following categories: (1) comforting or nurturing figures, (2) protective figures, (3) wisdom figures, and (4) comic relief figures. The helpers can be people from the client's life who are currently alive or those who have passed away, TV show characters, movie characters, book characters, celebrities, spiritual or religious leaders, pets, or animals. They cannot be inanimate objects. For instance, a special blanket may be a source of comfort, but it cannot serve as a comfort figure. The person, character, animal, etc. chosen for a particular category must have that characteristic. For example, the client must be able to imagine the protective qualities of a protective figure. Clients can repeat helpers in different categories, but when putting the helpers into a specific category, they must be able to envision the particular trait for the category.

If you are not certified in EMDR therapy, you can use guided imagery with the client. Instruct the client to visualize their current exposure therapy ladder step. The client should be able to get to a calm and relaxed state. Next, have the client describe the scene (where are they when accomplishing this task, what time of day it is, what they are wearing, etc.) and have them imagine working through the anxiety associated with the current step. Guided imagery will allow them to imagine overcoming their anxiety and accomplishing their current exposure ladder step, essentially serving as a mental rehearsal. If the client gets stuck or overwhelmed during the guided imagery, encourage the client to call on their team of helpers to get unstuck.

As with many clients with lifelong vaginismus I have worked with, I used a "future template" application of EMDR with Siobhan to help her to overcome her phobic anxiety of penetration. At each exposure therapy step when Siobhan felt stuck, we used EMDR and had her imagine confronting her anxiety about the step and completing the step successfully. This application served as a form of exposure therapy for Siobhan and helped her to build her confidence. In Noemi's case, we used the standard "past template" to target both her past sexual assault and her traumatic birth experience. Each memory took about three to five EMDR sessions to process. Noemi noted a significantly decrease in her PTSD symptoms after completing the series of EMDR sessions. With her trauma symptoms no longer interfering with her daily functioning, the course of therapy could then focus on her pelvic/sexual pain disorder. For Rebecca, the stand "past template" was also used to target her traumatic childhood memories, skiing accident, and resulting medical trauma. Because of Rebecca's chronic and complex childhood abuse, several months of EMDR therapy sessions were conducted, although she noticed important insights and important shifts after completing each memory. For Paula, the standard "past template" was used to target memories of grooming and sexual abuse, as well as retraumatizing events surrounding the trial. Paula reported a significant decline in both obsessive-compulsive disorder symptoms and PTSD symptoms after completing 12 sessions of EMDR therapy.

Another use for EMDR when working with clients with pelvic/sexual pain is for chronic pain management. A randomized controlled study in Spain compared the outcomes of patients with chronic pain who were given treatment as usual with those who received EMDR in addition to the treatment as usual. Data points were taken before treatment, immediately after treatment, and three months after treatment completion. The EMDR group received 12 individual 90-minute EMDR sessions over three months in which participants used EMDR to process both traumatic memories and memories that involved their pain symptoms. Immediately after treatment, the EMDR group demonstrated significantly less pain intensity, improved quality of life, and improved anxiety and depressive symptoms compared with the treatment-as-usual group. The EMDR group mostly maintained these positive gains at the three-month follow-up (Suárez et al., 2020).

## Incorporating the Partner Into Treatment

If a client is partnered, it is always helpful to incorporate the partner. In terms of what the research tells us about partners of women with pelvic/sexual pain disorders, historically it was hypothesized that male partners of women with vaginismus were passive and unassertive (Lahaie et al., 2010). However, when personality differences of male partners of women with vaginismus are compared with control participants or norms, there were no personality differences. And while some men who have partners with pelvic/sexual pain disorders experience erectile dysfunction or premature ejaculation, it appears to be secondary to vaginismus and its treatment (Reissing et al., 1999).

There is a dearth of research regarding women who are partnered with women who have pelvic/sexual pain disorders. Of the research that does exist regarding heterosexual couples in which the female partner has vaginismus, the research suggests that these relationships are strong, and partners are usually quite satisfied. In Tuğrul and Kabakci's (1997) study of 40 couples with vaginismus, 90% of husbands and 80% of wives evaluated their marriages as satisfactory (Davis & Reissing, 2007). In addition, several scholars have reported that couples with vaginismus have better relationship adjustment and communication compared with couples with other female sexual dysfunctions (Hawton & Catalan, 1990; Lahaie et al., 2010; Reissing et al., 1999).

For women with pelvic/sexual pain disorders, research supports the involvement of the partner in therapy. Strong communication, support by the partner, empathy demonstrated by the partner, and spiritual confidentiality were associated with positive outcomes in women with endometriosis who have painful intercourse. This study also compared couples with approach goals or goals focused on a positive outcome with couples with avoidance goals or goals that attempted to avoid a negative outcome. Results found that couples with approach goals experienced greater relationship and sexual satisfaction, highlighting the need for women with endometriosis to have their partners involved in treatment and urged for a holistic management approach of this disease (McKay et al., 2021).

Once the treatment plan has been established with the client, I find it helpful to ask their partner to attend one session. The goal of this session is to explain the treatment plan to the partner and answer any questions the partner may have. Many clients feel relieved about having their partner attend as many struggle with how to explain, for instance, the purpose of "taking sex off the table." Typically, once male partners understand the purpose of officially taking sex off the table (to remove the pressure and focus on rebuilding emotional and sexual intimacy outside of penetrative sex until the partner with the pelvic/sexual pain disorder gets medical clearance to proceed with penetrative sex), they are usually able to get on board with the treatment plan.

If a client's partner is resistant to the plan and wants to continue having sex with their partner despite the pain, this is a red flag for abuse in the relationship. Little to no progress can be made if abuse is ongoing in the relationship. If the client is in an abusive relationship, the therapeutic work needs to shift to this issue, and the pelvic/sexual pain disorder becomes secondary work. In addition, if you suspect abuse in the relationship after meeting with the partner, the partner should not be invited to any other therapy sessions. If the couple requests couples therapy or if there are issues other than the impact of the pelvic/sexual pain disorder that the couple wants to work on, I refer them out to couples' therapy.

In approaching treatment more holistically, Schultz et al. (2005) contend that it is important for the woman and her partner to decide what kind of treatment they would like to engage in and realize that they are both responsible for this choice. In tune with this sentiment, I ask each partner in the relationship to take ownership of their behaviors and that both partners are responsible for the choices they make around treatment. For instance, if a client and her partner agree that physical therapy and dilator therapy make sense in terms of treatment, the partner without the pelvic/sexual pain disorder can still help by taking on more of the household labor so the partner with pelvic/sexual pain can attend physical therapy and make time to do the dilator therapy.

I also talk to couples regarding the research about "response styles," or the partner's reaction to their partner's perceived pain and fear. Response styles of partners have been studied in couples with various chronic pain conditions. Response styles include (1) facilitative, (2) negative, and (3) solicitous. It has been suspected that couples with sexual pain use a solicitous response style, which enables couples to collude, avoid sexual interactions, and avoid treatment (Davis & Reissing, 2007). Similarly, a study of 354 women with provoked vestibulodynia found that partner pain catastrophizing was associated with solicitous partner responses and higher patient pain and depressive symptoms (Davis et al., 2015). Given this research, it is important that clients and their partners understand the difference between these styles and begin to practice facilitative responses.

Another useful goal when bringing in the partner for a session is developing broad and pleasure-focused intimate experiences. In helping clients and their partners to reach this goal, I often implore the "sexual menu exercise." Even for couples without pelvic/sexual pain, over the course of a long-term relationship, there will be points when penetrative sex is not an option. Other than a pelvic/sexual pain condition, common reasons why couples sometimes take a break from penetrative sex include when a partner is receiving treatment for a significant health issue such as cancer or having an autoimmune disease flare-up, when a partner is dealing with a traumatic experience, when a partner is postpartum, or when a partner is undergoing fertility treatment. Couples that have an expansive sexual repertoire find that there are many pleasurable and intimate ways to sexually connect other than penetrative sex. They are more able to adjust their sexual connection and maintain this connection even during difficult times. During the "sexual menu exercise," I ask couples to collaboratively create a sexual menu based on the following categories (Figure 7.4):

*Items always on the menu:* This category refers to physical activities that are almost always available to the couple and except in times of major crisis are enjoyable. This category could include physically intimate activities that are not overtly sexual. Common activities include holding hands, cuddling in bed, exchanging massages, taking a bath or shower together, or kissing on the neck or cheek.

*Seasonal items:* Just like the name implies, these are sexual menu items that are "seasonally" available or are occasionally available. This category includes activities that one partner may not prefer but the other partner really enjoys, so these activities happen only once in a while. For example, some partners really enjoy receiving oral sex but are with a partner who does not particularly enjoy giving oral sex. The partner who does not love giving oral sex may occasionally decide to make the effort for their partner's enjoyment, but it is not an activity the couple regularly partakes in.

*Weekly specials:* These sexual menu items become available due to a change in situation or environment. For instance, for many of my clients managing a pelvic/sexual pain condition, penetrative sex in certain positions or even certain outercourse activities may only be available when they are not in a flare-up of symptoms. Some women with endometriosis notice less pain at certain points in their menstrual cycle, which then makes penetrative sex a possible option. Similarly, other clients managing chronic health issues, including pelvic/sexual pain disorders and autoimmune diseases, or those undergoing treatment for cancer, usually need to contend with issues related to energy levels. The days or weeks they're feeling better, they may be open to more physically demanding sexual activities versus the weeks when they're feeling more drained.

*Amuse bouche:* This term refers to a pre-appetizer and means "a little taste." At high-end restaurants, visitors are often served an "amuse-bouche" before their appetizers. The serving size could be as small as one spoonful. Drawing parallels from this term, intimate activities

# Sexual Menu Exercise

## Regular Items

Activities that are always
generally comfortable and enjoyable

## Daily/Weekly Specials

Activities that become an option
due to a change

## Seasonal Items

Activities that are on rare
occasion okay to engage in

## Amuse-Bouche

Activities that are "a little taste"
- a lesser version of another activity

that fall under this category are sexual activities that someone may engage in for just a small amount of time or sexual activities they may need to modify to make less intense. In the earlier example in which one partner does not like to give oral sex, perhaps they can sometimes offer an "amuse-bouche" version – just briefly incorporating oral sex into the sexual experience. Certain positions may be too difficult or exhausting for those dealing with a pelvic/sexual pain or chronic health issue. However, couples could think about how the position could be modified or simply shorten the amount of time they engage in the activity. In terms of modification, many clients find certain outercourse sexual activities easily able to partake in with the right kind of physical support (OhNut, sitting in a chair, using pillows or a bolster, etc.).

For clients and their partners who seem hesitant about this exercise, help them to generate ideas for each category in session. Encourage clients and their partners to be very specific. There are many ways to kiss, let alone be touched or touch your partner. If stuck, ask clients and their partner to imagine a 30-second film clip of what they are envisioning and then describe that. Ask clients to consider the time of day when adding intimate activities to their sexual menu. Due to energy levels and living with the consequences of pelvic/sexual pain, certain activities may only be available in the morning, for instance, or only after a good night of sleep. Logistical issues such as when children might be in the home can also influence what time clients prefer for a certain sexual activity. Reviewing the sexual menu exercise is also another opportunity to provide psychoeducation about toys that can enhance pleasure and add variation to nonpenetrative sexual activities. The sexual menu is developed over time, and clients and their partners should continue to add and revise their menu.

Another common time I invite a partner to return to therapy is when the client is physically and emotionally ready to transition to penetrative sex. Just as any other step in this process, the transition back to penetrative sex is a scaffolded experience. Together with the partner, we identify conditions for success, which often include feeling emotionally connected to one another, not being pressed for time, having privacy, feeling well rested, etc. It is important that both the client and her partner understand that although they are transitioning back to penetrative sex, these experiences will feel rather clinical for the time being. The partner with pelvic/sexual pain will need to pre-dilate before any attempts at penetrative sex. For the first several attempts, the couple should simply "park the car," meaning the woman inserts the man's penis and allows him to stay inside for one minute with no thrusting. Not sexy but critical in building confidence. If the woman does not experience any pain with "parking the car," the couple can then try insertion with a few thrusts. From there, if there is no pain, the couple can continue to increase thrusting and overall penetrative time. I highly encourage couples to keep penetrative time to no longer than two to five minutes.

It is also important to prepare couples for what to do if there is pain during penetration, especially for those with living with chronic pelvic/sexual pain that may have flare-ups of symptoms. Remind couples that the focus should be on pleasure, not penetration, and encourage them to refer to their sexual menu if they are feeling stuck or limited in terms of what they can engage in sexually. I ask them to identify how they can shift in the moment to outercourse or another intimate activity like taking a shower together. I also like to highlight all the progress the woman with the pelvic/sexual pain condition has made, as well as the couple overall during this session.

## Important Takeaways

- Effective treatment involves a multimodal approach and includes collaboration with other healthcare professionals.
- Helping the client to establish an effective treatment team is imperative for progress and will require more effort upon the clinician's part.
- Treatment techniques found to be effective in treatment pelvic/sexual pain and trauma include graduated exposure therapy, psychoeducation, CBT, mindfulness techniques, EMDR therapy, and behavioral sex therapy interventions.

## References

Bergeron, S., Corsini-Munt, S., Aerts, L., Rancourt, K., & Rosen, N. O. (2015). Female sexual pain disorders: A review of the literature on etiology and treatment. *Current Sexual Health Reports, 7*, 159–169.

Brotto, L. A., Basson, R., Smith, K. B., Driscoll, M., & Sadownik, L. (2015). Mindfulness-based group therapy for women with provoked vestibulodynia. *Mindfulness, 6*, 417–432.

Brotto, L. A., Young, P., Smith, K. B., & Sadownik, L. A. (2015). Impact of a multidisciplinary vulvodynia program on sexual functioning and dyspareunia. *The Journal of Sexual Medicine, 12*, 238–247.

Bullo, S., & Weckesser, A. (2021). Addressing challenges in endometriosis pain communication between patients and doctors: The role of language. *Frontiers in Global Women's Health, 2*. https://doi.org/10.3389/fgwh.2021.764693

Burns, D. D. (1999). *The feeling good handbook*. Penguin.

Davis, H., & Reissing, E. (2007). Relationship adjustment and dyadic interaction in couples with sexual pain disorders: A critical review of the literature. *Sexual and Relationship Therapy, 22*, 245–254. doi:10.1080/14681990601026601

Davis, S. N., Bergeron, S., Sadikaj, G., Corsini-Munt, S., & Steben, M. (2015). Partner behavioral responses to pain mediate the relationship between partner pain cognitions and pain outcomes in women with provoked vestibulodynia. *The Journal of Pain, 16*(6), 549–557. doi:10.1016/j.jpain.2015.03.002

Hawton, K., & Catalan, J. (1990). Sex therapy for vaginismus: Characteristics of couples and treatment outcome. *Sexual and Marital Therapy, 5*, 39–48. doi:10.1080/02674659008407995

Lahaie, M., Boyer, S., Amsel, R., Khalifé, S., & Binik, Y. (2010). Vaginismus: A review of the literature on the classification/diagnosis, etiology and treatment. *Women's Health, 6*, 705–719. doi:10.2217/whe.10.46

Masheb, R. M., Kerns, R. D., Lozano, C., Minkin, M. J., & Richman, S. (2009). A randomized clinical trial for women with vulvodynia: Cognitive-behavioral therapy vs. supportive therapy. *Pain, 141*, 31–40.

McKay, C. L., Van Niekerk, L. M., & Matthewson, M. L. (2021). An exploration of dyadic relationship approach-avoidance goals and relationship and sexual satisfaction in couples coping with endometriosis. *Archives of Sexual Behavior.* https://doi.org/10.1007/s10508-021-02150-1

Parnell, L. (2008). *Tapping in: A step-by-step guide to activating your healing resources through bilateral stimulation: An EMDR-related technique.* Sounds True.

Parnell, L. (2013). *Attachment-focused EMDR: Healing relational trauma.* W. W. Norton & Company.

Reissing, E., Binik, Y., & Khalifé, S. (1999). Does vaginismus exist? A critical review of the literature. *The Journal of Nervous & Mental Disease, 187*, 261–274. http://ovidsp.tx.ovid.com.ezproxy.bu.edu/sp-3.13.1a/ovidweb.cgi

Schultz, W., Basson, R., Binik, Y., Eschenbach, D., Wesselmann, U., & Lankveld, J. (2005). Women's sexual pain and its management. *The Journal of Sexual Medicine, 2*, 301–316. doi:10.1111/j.1743-6109.2005.20347.x

Shapiro, F. (2014). *Getting past your past: Take control of your life with self-help techniques from EMDR therapy*. Rodale.

Shapiro, F. (2018). *Eye movement desensitization and reprocessing (EMDR) therapy: Basic principles, protocols, and procedures*. The Guilford Press.

Shapiro, F., & Forrest, M. S. (2016). *EMDR: The breakthrough therapy for overcoming anxiety, stress, and trauma*. Basic Books.

Shapiro, F., Kaslow, F. W., & Maxfield, L. (2007). *Handbook of EMDR and family therapy processes*. John Wiley & Sons.

Suárez, N. A., Pérez, J. M., Redolar-Ripoll, D., Hogg, B. M., Gardoki-Souto, I., Guerrero, F. G., Cabrera, S. J., Bernal, D. S., Amann, B. L., & Moreno-Alcázar, A. (2020). EMDR versus treatment-as-usual in patients with chronic non-malignant pain: A randomized controlled pilot study. *Journal of EMDR Practice and Research, 14*(4), 190–205. https://doi.org/10.1891/emdr-d-20-00004

Tuğrul, C., & Kabakci, E. (1997). Vaginismus and its correlates. *Sexual and Marital Therapy, 12*(1), 23–34. https://doi.org/10.1080/02674659708408199

# 8

## CASE VIGNETTES – ASSESSMENT AND TREATMENT

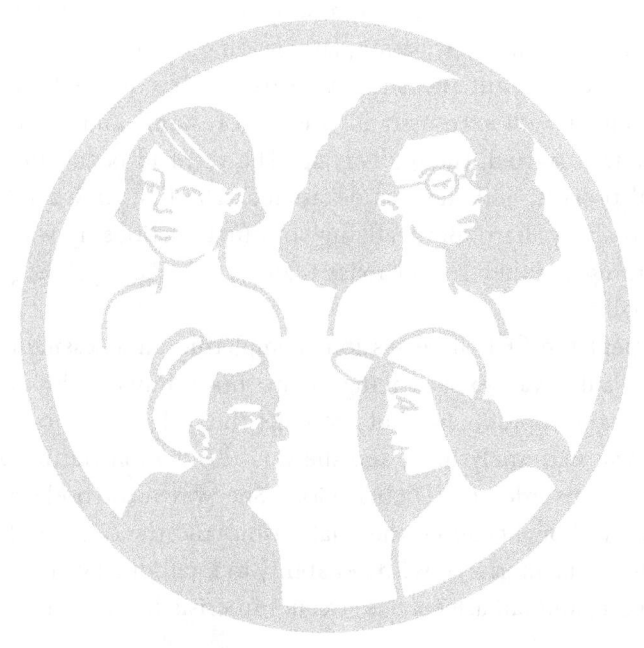

DOI: 10.4324/9781003168232-8

## Paula

"I really thought we were going to be together . . . now I can see that was never his intention . . . just part of the game. I feel like a moron," Paula stated in session the week her case had started trial. Of all the types of trauma cases clinicians work with, I find working with victims of grooming abuse particularly painful. Many trauma survivors seek therapy at a time when they know they have been wronged. But those who have experienced grooming abuse initially present "trauma bonded" to their perpetrator and label the experience as "my first relationship" or "my first love," just like Paula did. They may enter therapy knowing in their gut that something about the situation was off but are usually still coming out of the fog of years of abuse. Working with clients like Paula is sort of like watching a horror movie in which you already know the ending, and it's a bad one. You must watch in suspense, patiently yet full of dread, as you watch the main character put the pieces of the horror together. As a clinician, managing your own reactions to these situations can sometimes be challenging.

Paula entered therapy due to distress around her "first relationship," which had evolved over several years during high school years with a teacher/coach. She had disclosed to a mandated reporter the year prior, which triggered an investigation, later leading to a criminal case against her teacher/coach. Initially, she was heartbroken, confused, disoriented, and presented with extremely high levels of shame and self-blame. But once the trial started, the gig was up. The veil had been lifted through the legal process, and she was devastated. The first time a relationship ends, it is always hard. But realizing your first relationship was just years of grooming and then sexual abuse is an earthquake psychologically and emotionally.

We spent the first three sessions completing an assessment and full history. Paula was experiencing many posttraumatic stress disorder (PTSD)–like symptoms but did not meet the full criteria for PTSD. Her anxiety was extremely high, and she was also demonstrating obsessive-compulsive disorder (OCD) behaviors. She was most bothered by her ruminating thoughts about the relationship and the ongoing legal case. These thoughts interfered with her ability to focus during class, complete schoolwork, and fall asleep. She was not in crisis but was close to it.

Paula reported growing up in a suburban community of a large East Coast city. She was the second oldest of four girls, all of whom attended a private all-girls Christian school from kindergarten through high school. Both of her parents were professionals who worked full-time, but they had a lot of extended family living nearby who often helped with shuttling the girls to their various after school activities. Paula reported having overall a happy childhood – she did not have any health issues, she felt close with her family, she had close friends, she excelled in science, and she was a top soccer player in the region. She did not fit the stereotypical image of a teen who would be vulnerable to grooming and sexual abuse. But that is part of the point – anyone can be vulnerable to this type of abuse.

### Understanding the Grooming Process

Grooming refers to behaviors that an adult abuser uses to desensitize or prepare a child or teen for sexual abuse. Grooming is a slow process and may occur over a period of years, as it did in Paula's case. Later in treatment when we started to talk about the grooming process, she exclaimed,

> I don't even know when I would say it started. . . . Was it him befriending my parents, the other girls' parents so they would trust him? Was it when he would touch my foot trying to teach me a different technique for kicking? Was it when he started to text me . . . about soccer, about the other girls in the class? Asking me to show him the two different uniforms the team captains were choosing between?

Grooming occurs in distinct phases. Over the course of therapy, Paula came to understand and identify how the grooming process occurred in her situation:

1.  *The introduction:* Adult abuser meets child victim. Often perpetrators have some access to children due to their career or social standing. Examples include religious leaders like a priest, a teacher, a tutor, a coach, or a doctor. Adult abusers are often well-respected

and well-liked members of the community. Parents or other adults believe the perpetrator has a skill or guidance to give to the child and therefore misread the intentions when an adult abuser takes interest in their child. Paula's perpetrator was both a teacher and a coach, allowing him access to her as well as many other teens. He was a well-liked by both the girls and their families from the school where he taught.

2.   *A special relationship is formed:* The abuser takes special interest in the victim, often promising the child and their family some sort of benefit from the relationship. A full two years before the sexual abuse started, Paula's perpetrator offered to provide her with one-on-one private coaching to take her soccer skills to "the next level." As Paula explained, "I desperately wanted to play in college, but neither of my parents were athletes, so my parents were thrilled that he offered to coach me with some one-on-one sessions." Other common examples are priests offering a child and/or their family a special role within the church or teachers offering to spend extra time and attention after school with a particular child. The child or teen is made to feel special by the abuser and may genuinely benefit from what the abuser has to offer, as often the family does. The special relationship may exist for months or even years before any overt inappropriate behavior occurs. The child and adult abuser grow closer in their "special" relationship. Many adult survivors recall feeling that the perpetrator was as close as a "father," "older brother," "cousin," "aunt," etc. The special relationship may even extend to the entire family, and other family members may receive additional attention and favors. This enables the abuser to gain the trust of not only the victim but also of anyone who could spot the abuse and possibly intervene on behalf of the victim. If the abuser can win over the family, this only makes it more difficult for the child victim to ever disclose the sexual abuse. After processing the sexual abuse, Paula realized part of what kept her trapped in the secrecy of what was happening was that she thought no one would believe her because he was so well-liked by everyone. Or that somehow it was her fault because, again, he was so well-liked.

3.   *Boundaries are blurred:* Eventually, a boundary will be violated, but first the abuser desensitizes the child or teen victim to inappropriate

behaviors. Usually, the first boundaries violated are not physical. For instance, the adult abuser may insist on the child's telling him/her a secret, or the adult abuser may start disclosing intimate details about their own life. These intimate details may include information about their dating life, a sexual story about themselves or someone else, or even their own struggles with a work conflict or family conflict. Paula stated that she and her teacher/coach became closer over her sophomore year of high school and talked about "all kinds of deep stuff. I really viewed him like a friend or brother." Physical touching is likely already occurring but may not be overtly inappropriate. Paula noted that over sophomore year, high fiving eventually evolved to hugging and then to playful pushing and swatting and that he occasionally would even play with her hair, always, of course, when others were not around. Some adult survivors recall feeling uncomfortable but unsure how to handle the situation, especially when other adults witnessed the boundary crossings and did nothing (often this is because the family and community members were groomed by the perpetrator, too!). Others recall the escalation of behaviors being so subtle that they did not remember feeling alarmed and only now as an adult are able to recognize the inappropriate pattern unfolding. Both are common experiences.

4.   *A violation occurs:* By the time a clear sexual boundary is crossed, the child or teen victim is so desensitized or feels so powerless and trapped by the relationship they do not know what to do. The sexual contact may even be wanted by the child or teen victim, but this is a product of the grooming. Because of the slow progression of behaviors leading to the abuse, the child victim is unable to see the adult abuser for what they are – the only one responsible for the abuse. By the time sexual contact starts occurring, the child victim is so emotionally close to the perpetrator that they do not believe they can end the abuse. The abusing adult often frames the sexual abuse as an extension of their special relationship, making the child victim feel confused. Paula viewed her relationship with the teacher/coach as an actual romantic relationship. He even told her that once she graduated high school, they would be able to tell their friends and family about the relationship.

5.   *The aftermath:* The sexual abuse may occur just a few times, or it could continue for years, even extending into adulthood. Because the adult abuser usually also has a relationship with the victim's family and friends, it makes it almost impossible for the child or teen victim to break away from the adult abuser. An adult survivor I once worked with explained that she confronted her abuser and begged him to stop visiting her family. The perpetrator continued to email both of her parents, continued to make plans with her family, and even continued to set up mentoring appointments to meet with the teen victim through her parents. Unfortunately, these are common stories. Paula recalled how in her senior year of high school, she wanted to "break up" with her teacher/coach, but he was relentless in pursuing her, and she started to not see a way out of the situation until she moved away for college. Through the grooming process, perpetrators make the child victim believe they also wanted the sexual contact, which is one of the reasons these crimes go widely unreported. Furthermore, the adult abuser's social standing and social power make the victim believe no one would believe them anyway if they were to report the crime.

### "But Why is Sex Hurting More Now?"

As part of my assessment, I ask about past and current relationships, as well as the sexual dynamics of these relationships. Paula was comfortable discussing her sexual pain early in therapy. Something particularly distressing to Paula was the fact that she had pain during penetrative sex with the perpetrator but was now experiencing even worse pain with her current partner. Paula stated she felt safe with her current partner and did not believe the pain was related to any current relationship conflict or distress. It is likely that the stress related to the abuse and ongoing legal case had contributed to a worsening of symptoms, especially if unconsciously Paula was guarding her pelvis. Upon any attempt at penetration, Paula experienced a burning sensation at the vaginal opening or vestibule. Paula had previously found pelvic exams painful and was also having difficulty inserting tampons. Paula had previously told her OB/GYN about the pain but was dismissed. Playing soccer with a pad was "less than ideal," as she explained it. I referred her to a pelvic pain specialist, who diagnosed her with vulvodynia and pelvic floor muscle dysfunction.

Pacing is key. Each client will approach the pace at which they want to address or treat their pelvic/sexual pain problem differently. Despite going through the legal proceedings regarding her sexual abuse, playing soccer for her university, and taking a rigorous science curriculum, Paula was motivated to address her pelvic/sexual pain. Paula admitted she was motivated by wanting to please her partner and a desire to "feel normal." In Paula's view, having pain with sex as a college-aged woman was just another way she was different from her peers. She said, "Having your teacher be your first boyfriend is bad enough."

Therapeutic work with Paula was a delicate balance between helping her to process her "first relationship," which she later came to view as abusive, and addressing current stressors such as the consequences of the ongoing legal proceedings and her pelvic/sexual pain. In many ways, addressing the pelvic/sexual pain allowed Paula to feel in control of some aspect of her life, as the legal proceedings were out of her control. Early on in treatment we worked on assertiveness skills, something she identified as needing in many areas of her life. Paula's treatment team included myself, a psychiatrist, a pelvic floor physical therapist, and an OB/GYN specialist. Together we encouraged Paula to communicate assertively with us and let her determine the pace of her treatment. In Paula's case specifically, it was extremely important that she communicate with her treatment team about when she was feeling too triggered or overwhelmed by the legal proceedings to engage in internal physical therapy work.

The discovery process in preparation of determining the specific criminal charges was particularly distressing for Paula. It was in this process that the illusion of her "first relationship" faded and she saw the sinister nature of what had occurred. Her PTSD-like symptoms, anxiety, and OCD behaviors became extremely high. I discussed with Paula the option of doing eye movement desensitization and reprocessing (EMDR) therapy but explained it was imperative for her to consult with her lawyer. Although the choice is always ultimately the client's, sometimes lawyers do not want clients to undergo EMDR therapy until a trial is complete if there is a need to demonstrate a certain level of distress. The prosecution team reassured Paula that they did not believe Paula experiencing a relief in symptoms would impact their case. Paula chose to undergo EMDR therapy. In total, we completed 12 EMDR sessions, which centered on three of the most upsetting traumatic memories about the abuse. Paula experienced a significant decrease in her symptoms because of EMDR therapy.

Once her case went to trial, the anger of what had happened set in. I often notice that once clients are no longer in the crisis of dealing with PTSD symptoms, the anger over what occurred finally has the space to emerge. Fueling this anger was also being the target of online bullying by her some of her former classmates who made immature, but nevertheless painful, accusations against her (being a "slut," "teacher's pet," "out for money"). The bullying eventually ceased once her perpetrator was found guilty, but the damage was already done. Paula's parents made the difficult decision to relocate the family out of state because they, too, felt angry about the lack of support from the surrounding community. The focus of therapy then shifted to help Paula process her emotional reactions towards the trial ending and developing healthy strategies for expressing her anger.

## Violet

Violet was a self-referred client who sought therapy for her anxiety and chronic pelvic/sexual pain due to endometriosis. During our assessment, Violet explained her family history was "somewhat of a soap opera." Violet's mother was white and had her at age 20 as a single mother. She learned later in her teen years that her father was black, was significantly older than her mother, was married with children, and was also an established professional in the area. As a young adult, Violet attempted to contact her father and her other siblings but was told to "back off." Violet later did an ancestry test, and an online database connected her with another half-sibling from her father. She developed a relationship with this brother, who was also the product of an affair and had also been rejected from their father's family.

"I was a biracial child who grew up in a 'white-trash' family. And my mom was a true single mother – she never got a dollar from my dad or an hour of childcare help. But honestly, despite this, I have happy memories of my childhood," Violet said when asked about her childhood. Violet lived with her mother, her mother's parents, and various siblings of her mother (some who were close in Violet's age). Violet stated she always had someone to play with and watch over her. Her mother received her GED and then her associate degree to become a medical assistant. When Violet was five years old, her mom started to date her stepfather. They married when Violet was seven, moved into their own home, and soon after had two children of their own. She remembered her mom and stepfather trying to get her excited about having her own room at their new house, but not living with her grandparents was a difficult adjustment. Her first memories of anxiety symptoms were during this adjustment period.

Violet began her period at 13 and soon after began to experience significant pain with her period, as well as heavy bleeding. Both her mother and doctor told her that this was a normal part of womanhood and that she would have to find a way to cope with the pain. She stated that her symptoms grew progressively worse each year and impacted her ability to focus on her studies and participate in extracurricular activities. Violet reported deep pain with penetration with her first sexual partner in high school and later in college some bleeding after penetrative sex. "I just figured I probably had some kind of horrible cancer that no one would figure out until I was on my death bed," Violet lamented one session. Over the years, she had been to multiple specialists for her symptoms and had heard various explanations about her symptoms, including needing to lose weight, having a tilted uterus, having a low pain tolerance, etc.

Violet attended a local state university on a partial scholarship to study early childhood education. Violet stated that her endometriosis symptoms continued to worsen during this time, and she often missed days of class when she had her period. During college, Violet reported beginning to question her sexuality and began to identify as bisexual. However, as she explained, "I was always doubting myself. I've always felt like I didn't really know who I was – probably because there has always been some part of me that has literally been rejected by other people." She felt her existence was denied by her father and his family, she felt rejected by both black and white peers due to her biracial identity, she felt dismissed by doctors for her pelvic/sexual pain symptoms, and then she experienced bi-erasure from her peers and family. It was no wonder she doubted herself after experiencing a sexual assault by a friend in college.

"We had been friends since freshmen year . . . we certainly had drunk many times together before . . . not sure why that time was different," Violet said about the night of the sexual assault. She vividly remembered saying "no" when he started trying to kiss her. Things escalated from there. They avoided each other after that night, which made Violet feel guilty, as if she had done something wrong. Violet initially did not tell anyone about the sexual assault because she did not think anyone would believe her or that it would be chalked up to a miscommunication after a night of heavy drinking. It still bothered her, though. Eventually, she disclosed the assault to the college administration, but it was ignored due to the drinking being involved.

After graduation, Violet worked in a private religious school as a teacher, but she realized she would never be able to afford to live on the salary. She lived back at home with her mom and stepdad, waitressed a few nights a week after work, and decided to send out some graduate school applications for a master's degree in education. After living in Tennessee her entire life, she decided for graduate school she'd like try living somewhere else. To her delight and her family's disappointment, she was accepted to her reach school in a large East Coast city. "I thought I would fit in better in a big East Coast city – and actually that's been mostly true." She even finally got a doctor to investigate her symptoms.

"I would spend a few days vomiting and completely unable to move from the pain when I got my period by the time I had moved. It was my new primary care doctor that finally said, 'This is not normal' and referred me to an endometriosis specialist in the city." At 26, nearly 13 years after her first symptoms, Violet finally underwent surgery, which confirmed extensive endometriosis and required one of her ovaries to be removed. Coming out of the haze of the anesthesia, she remembered being simultaneously relieved to finally have a diagnosis and devastated after hearing she would likely not be able to have children. "I also thought the surgery was a cure – no one told me otherwise," Violet later reflected when discussing how difficult it still was to manage this systemic disease.

Upon entering treatment Violet's biggest concern was managing her anxiety. While she was not having full-blown panic attacks, her baseline daily anxiety was quite high. After the assessment, Violet realized her anxiety was being driven by multiple life stressors, including (1) her ongoing pelvic/sexual pain and other endometriosis symptoms, (2) financial instability, (3) professional burnout, and (4) experiencing distress and confusion about her sexual orientation. It was also clear from our assessment that Violet struggled deeply with trusting her judgement and believing in herself.

## Creating a Treatment Team Within the Realities of Life

Violet lacked an appropriate treatment team to manage and care for her endometriosis upon entering treatment. Since her surgery, she had not had any follow-up care and had relocated to the Philadelphia area for a new job. Like all clients, the types of resources available to Violet were driven by her finances. And like most Millennials, Violet was burdened by student debt, and her salary had not kept up with the cost of living. The illusion of teaching being a stable and fulfilling job had faded the past few years despite her best efforts to change what was in her control, like the type of school she taught for. It was in our conversations about creating a treatment team that Violet tearfully acknowledged wanting to leave teaching but felt trapped by her student debt and degree, which she believed to be useless outside of a school setting.

Until she decided her next steps for her career, we had to work within the confines of her current health insurance plan, which was an extremely limited HMO. After learning more about endometriosis treatment, Violet wanted to undergo an excision surgery. However, this procedure is typically not covered by insurance. Out-of-pocket this surgery would cost Violet $15,000, if not more. She felt devastated, and I encouraged her to focus on the components of her treatment that she could control. We agreed to focus on her most bothersome physical symptoms which Violet identified being her fatigue, urinary urgency, and pelvic pain.

Violet agreed to sign a release of information to allow me to help with coordinating care through her OB/GYN. After speaking with her OB/GYN, she agreed to write a script for pelvic floor physical therapy, although Violet's options were very limited due to the HMO. After finding a pelvic floor physical therapist who accepted her health insurance, we consulted with the physical therapist together via phone on strategies about how to get the most out of her 10 approved sessions, including teaching physical therapy exercises that could be done at home and spacing out her appointments more so she could be seen over a longer period time. Luckily, the physical therapist was eventually able to secure more appointments for Violet due to the extent of pelvic floor muscle dysfunction she was experiencing.

Violet expressed interest in wanting to see a dietician after learning that both interstitial cystitis (IC) and endometriosis symptoms can sometimes be reduced with dietary changes. It was, however, another moment of being disappointed in the lack of follow-up care postsurgery but also an opportunity for her now to gain more control over managing her health. Violet's insurance did cover three appointments with a dietician, but we struggled finding someone who accepted her insurance who also had knowledge about dietary recommendations for IC and endometriosis. The pelvic floor physical therapist connected Violet to a dietician she knew who was experienced with these conditions, but she did not accept insurance. As a compromise, the dietician agreed to slide her fee for Violet and offered shorter appointments spread over a longer period, which made these appointments more affordable for her. Over a span of several months, they worked together on implementing the low-oxalate diet for IC and an anti-inflammatory diet to help with the endometriosis. After doing her own research on chronic pain management, Violet also reported wanting to try acupuncture. Unfortunately, Violet's HMO did not cover this type of treatment. However, there was a community clinic that had acupuncture clinicians in training who could offer sliding scale fees.

Violet's case highlights the reality for many of our clients who may have limited financial resources. Clinicians who decide to become specialists in pelvic/sexual pain need to connect with the other healthcare professionals in their communities who treat clients with these disorders. These other professionals can become amazing resources and help to come up with creative solutions when financial barriers become an issue. The other reality for women like Violet is that there is no cure for her conditions. However, the goal was effective management of these conditions to enable her to live the most fulfilling life possible. Violet was able to see notable improvements in her chronic pelvic pain and urinary symptoms through this multimodal treatment approach.

One year after the start of counseling and creating her treatment team, Violet no longer needed pelvic floor physical therapy but continued both internal and external physical therapy interventions at home. She also knew what physical signs would indicate that she may need to return to pelvic floor physical therapy. She now understood the mind–body connection and how stress played a role in the flare-up of her symptoms, thus making stress management an important component to her long-term care. Violet no longer needed to meet with the dietician and had made several dietary modifications that helped reduce her pain and flare-ups. Violet still attended acupuncture every other week at the community clinic as the treatment seemed to significantly reduce her chronic pain and fatigue.

## Cultivating Self-Confidence

It was easy for Violet to doubt herself. Attempts by Violet to better understand herself and her identities were sadly met with rejection – first by her father and his family. She felt white-washed by her mother and her family. She struggled being biracial growing up in a mostly white community and was often left with the feeling of not belonging. Her endometriosis symptoms were dismissed by doctors for over a decade, leaving Violet doubtful that she even knew her own body. She struggled with her recollection of the sexual assault during college, which was also dismissed by authority figures at the school. In college, she began to explore her sexuality and identified as bisexual but began to question this after feedback from peers and people she dated. And to top it all off, as Violet explained, "I obviously didn't pick well in terms of a career that would allow me to meet my goal of becoming financially stable. Sure, I have a master's degree, but I am no better off than my mom once you factor in the student debt that I will never be able to get rid of."

Cultivating self-confidence was something needed in all areas of Violet's life, including how she managed her pelvic/sexual pain, approached dating, and made choices in her professional life. Her diagnosis with endometriosis and IC became an important reference point for her. It signified that she *did* know herself and she knew her body. Through therapy, Violet processed not only the medical gaslighting she experienced but also the reaction from her college when she reported the sexual assault. If she was right about her body, maybe she was also right about the sexual assault. She began to realize she could trust her judgement and that often it was not her judgement that failed her but rather authority figures in positions of power such as her father, her doctors, the college administrators, etc. Navigating the process of creating her treatment team and feeling more in control of her medical care provided opportunities for Violet to feel more confident as well.

Increasing her self-confidence seemed to help Violet relieve the pressure she had been putting on herself when it came to dating. She became less fixated on feeling like she needed to choose to date men or women. "If someone interests me, I'll date them. Beyond that I'm not going to let myself or other people try and force me into a particular label right now." As she began to feel more confident, she also became surer of the gut feeling she had been having for a few years that she needed to leave teaching.

## Rebecca

Even the way Rebecca sat in my office made her appear smaller and almost childlike, her shoulders curled in, her hair blocking her eyes, and her torso sunken into the sofa. She clutched a tissue, eyes to the ground, and began crying before the first session even began. "I don't really see the point in being here, to be honest," she explained. I did not know if she meant in therapy, on earth, or both, but my gut reaction was alerting me to screen for suicidality. "None of my doctors, my physical therapist, my husband, no one really, knows what to do with me at this point. Dr. Z told me he would only continue treating me if I saw you, so, here I am," she sniffled, slowly looking up at me. I always dread hearing these kinds of statements, as if psychotherapy is a panacea and by default I, the therapist, some sort of magician.

Rebecca was referred by her pelvic/sexual pain OB/GYN specialist and pelvic floor physical therapist for psychotherapy. Both noted an unexplained lack of progress after three years of working together and questioned whether a psychological component was hindering their medical treatment of their patient. About five years prior, Rebecca was involved in a serious accident while backcountry skiing in Utah with her husband. She dislocated a shoulder, broke one of her legs, and experienced a pelvic fracture that required surgery. Unfortunately, during the surgery Rebecca contracted a methicillin-resistant *Staphylococcus aureus* (MRSA) infection on her upper thighs and pelvis. "Between the pelvis fracture and the MRSA, I spent three months in the hospital. I was supposed to be transferred to a rehab, but my father, thank God, stepped in and paid for me to receive around-the-clock care at home for a few months," Rebecca noted. The details of the skiing accident and following medical treatment sounded traumatizing, yet she spoke about them in a depressed but very matter-of-fact way. Since the accident and the MRSA infection, Rebecca experienced chronic severe pelvic pain. She had received various diagnoses over the years, including vulvodynia, pelvic floor dysfunction, pudendal nerve entrapment, fibromyalgia, somatization disorder, etc. Rebecca reported feeling "totally hopeless," and it was understandable as to why. Over the past few years, she had tried a range of treatments, including "all kinds of injections, nerve blocks, a bunch of creams, physical therapy, an ultrasound wave therapy thing, pain meds, antidepressants. . . . I've tried it all, and there have been some improvements but not much."

"I don't see how this is related," Rebecca scoffed when I explained my rationale behind wanting to do a thorough history with her as part of my assessment. And as most therapists know, the clients who often dig in the most around the idea that their history isn't related to their current problems are the clients whose pasts are usually very much so connected to their current issues. "What does my f – – up pelvis have to do with my dead brother?" she snapped. Although this comment was unpleasant to be on the receiving end of as the therapist, it did reveal some fight left in her, which was a relief given how depressed she presented.

Rebecca was the third child of four to an upper middle class Jewish family living in the suburbs of New York City. Her father had a successful law practice in New York City, and her mother was a stay-at-home-mom while she and her siblings were young. When Rebecca was five years old, her brother Nathan, who was eight at the time, was diagnosed with childhood leukemia. After a two-year battle with leukemia, he passed away. She explained she had only a few memories of Nathan before he became ill. Once Nathan became ill, Rebecca and her two other brothers spent most of their time with their paternal grandparents. Her father worked long hours, and her mother spent most of her time back and forth from the hospital and caring for Nathan when he was at home. Rebecca said her paternal grandparents were "very sweet" but elderly and unable to manage her older brother Samuel's significant behavioral problems.

After Nathan's passing, Rebecca and her brothers returned to their parents' home full time but "my Dad escaped by working all of the time, and my mom was profoundly depressed and barely functioning. It was like living with a zombie. For the rest of elementary school, I got myself and my brother David ready for school. Half the time there wasn't even breakfast food in the house." And while her older brother Samuel "had always been off," he became physically and sexually abusive towards her. She and David mostly huddled together in one of their bedrooms, avoiding interacting with Samuel, who would hit them, push them, and expose himself to them. As they grew into pre-teens and teens, Samuel's behavior escalated. A few times, he grabbed Rebecca's hand and forced her to touch his penis. Other times he groped her. "As we grew, David seemed to get more of the physical abuse and I the sexual abuse. It was a shared hell, though. It is part of why we have always been so close," Rebecca noted.

She explained that school had become her own escape. At school she was safe and well-liked by her peers and teachers. She was smart and a hard worker, always receiving high grades and praises from the teachers. "They knew about my brother Nathan dying, and I think they suspected we were being neglected at home, so I got some extra attention from my teachers. I didn't mind. I needed to be doted on," Rebecca said. During the summers, she and David were sent to overnight camp for two months, providing another much-needed escape from the family home. The summers spent at camp helped to foster her love for the outdoors. Camp was also how she met her husband, Jacob. "He was a city boy and came from a more conservative family. We started dating my junior year of high school. He had already started college, so we saw each other only on the weekends. Regardless, it certainly was another nice get-away from my house." Rebecca said that at the end of high school, her parents separated and then divorced. She explained she was not surprised by this, as her mom "never recovered" after Nathan's passing, while her dad wanted to "still live his life." Her dad relocated to New York City to be closer to his law firm and new girlfriend. The marital home was sold, and her mom moved into a smaller home nearby with her and her brothers.

"A smaller home meant there was practically no space for David and me to even attempt to separate ourselves from my mom's depression and Samuel's abuse. Things got very bad. David eventually ran away and moved in with my dad and finished high school in the city. My out was getting married," Rebecca stated. Just out of high school, Rebecca and Jacob married and moved into family housing at his university. She began to take college classes at a local women's university. She described their early married life as loving and filled with "adventure," as they camped in the summers and skied in the winters on the weekends. The couple had waited until marriage to engage in sexual activity, and Rebecca reported no issues with penetrative sex and found sex to be pleasurable. She stated that after getting married, other than her brother David, she was rarely in contact with her parents and had never contacted Samuel again.

After college, Jacob was accepted into a doctoral program in England, where Rebecca worked as one of the administrative assistants in a department at the university. She loved their years spent abroad and explained that any free time they had was spent traveling. Her first pregnancy was a surprise, but she said they soon became excited and were thrilled to have a son, whom they named after Rebecca's brother, David. Three years later, at age 28, Rebecca had their daughter, Shira. She reported no issues during pregnancy or delivery. She did experience one miscarriage between her pregnancies. Rebecca reported that she and Jacob adjusted to being parents well but did experience a few years when their sexual frequency was "very low," which she attributed to the stress of raising a young family. Rebecca also suspected having possible postpartum depression after the birth of her daughter and acknowledged painfully reflecting on her own childhood during this time.

Eventually, the family returned stateside for Jacob's job, and Rebecca explained,

> We basically just went wherever Jacob could get a decent teaching job – We've lived in Colorado and then Utah for a few years, which we loved because of the close access to skiing and hiking. Then Jacob

was offered a tenure-track job back in the northeast, where we could be close to my brother David and some of his siblings . . . so we went.

Rebecca discussed the transition back to the Northeast and her focus on raising their children while David worked. Once the children were off to college, Rebecca began working as a paralegal. Rebecca explained that her adult life had been "pretty charmed, lovely, actually" up until her skiing accident.

### When the Body Becomes a Prison

After consulting with Rebecca's OB/GYN specialist and pelvic floor physical therapist during the assessment phase, I questioned my next steps in treatment. Both providers suspected some kind of "psychological block," even though Rebecca had never shared with either about her childhood. They also believed her nervous system was, as the physical therapist put it, "always ramped up – stuck in an overactive state." Both providers acknowledged being puzzled by Rebecca's lack of progress.

After the assessment, Rebecca and I discussed her therapy goals. "I don't really know, other than just wanting my pain to be lower. . . . I can't keep living like this," she said tearfully. Normally, I would go over an exposure therapy ladder with corresponding client goals, but I worried Rebecca would become too overwhelmed with this long-term planning. I attempted to introduce a few basic cognitive behavioral therapy (CBT) techniques, including the pain and anxiety scale, which failed miserably. "Everything feels the same – I don't know what to tell you," Rebecca remarked when I attempted the pain and anxiety scales with her.

Typically, I like clients to have established some CBT coping skills and other emotional regulation techniques before attempting EMDR therapy, but Rebecca's responses to the CBT skills indicated she was not in an emotional place to do the work required to benefit from CBT. I pitched the idea of using EMDR therapy to process the skiing accident and resulting medical trauma, as well as her childhood trauma. Although she doubted my theory that processing the trauma might help with her pelvic pain condition, to her credit, she was at least open to the idea. I explained if we could get her "nervous system unstuck from fight/flight/freeze mode," she may start to respond to the medical treatment of her pelvic pain differently.

We spent three sessions identifying specific traumatic childhood memories to process using EMDR therapy and creating a peaceful place and resource team for Rebecca to access during processing if needed. When processing traumatic memories with EMDR, it is advised to start with the earliest and/or worst memories, as memories that occurred later, which left the client feeling similarly, will likely be processed, too. Our first target memory was when Rebecca was about seven years old, about six months after Nathan's passing. She recalled needing to use the bathroom badly but being fearful to leave her room. She remembered checking the hallway to make sure Samuel was not there. Rebecca said the hallway was clear, so she made a run for it, when sudden Samuel came around the corner laughing and grabbed her by her shoulders and then inappropriately touched her. Rebecca stated that the image that represented the worst part of this memory was, "Being back in my room afterward, being alone, crying." The negative cognition associated with this memory was "I am powerless."

Almost 40 minutes into the EMDR session, Rebecca had a significant insight: "When I was a little girl, my house was a prison, and now my body is a prison. I am trapped." This statement revealed the connection between her childhood traumas and her pelvic pain disorder. It took seven EMDR sessions to process this single childhood traumatic memory, as it was linked to many other childhood traumas. As Rebecca progressed through the sessions she shifted from the belief of "I am powerless" to "I now have choices." Through the EMDR sessions, Rebecca became more aware of all the creative and brave ways both she and her brother David tried to manage a dangerous situation. "I got out. I found a way to escape," she reflected during one EMDR session, noting her involvement in extracurricular activities, overnight camp, spending excess time at friends' houses, and ultimately permanently exiting the home when she got married. This empowering realization made her question, "How do I get out now? How do I escape the pain?"

While we continued to process two other childhood memories and the skiing accident, a major shift had already occurred. I gently approached an idea with Rebecca that she had previously rejected – finding pleasure in the now, even with her current physical restrictions. I tried to reframe these experiences as her "outs," her "escapes" from the pain. With the help of the pelvic floor physical therapist, we collaboratively came up with a list of small physical activities Rebecca could engage in. Because of Rebecca's lifelong love of the outdoors, we also tried to incorporate opportunities to be outside. They were very small but accomplishable tasks, with the hope that she could enjoy an experience in her body. For instance, one activity was to walk to the end of driveway each day with her husband. Another was to lie on a blanket outside in the sun with her dog for 20 minutes. As Rebecca and I continued to process, the pelvic floor physical therapist and Rebecca continued to expand her physical activities.

Both myself and her other providers noticed an emotional and neurological shift. Rebecca seemed lighter, she smiled, she sat upright, she laughed, she looked us in the eyes, and she was reporting slightly less pain. In tune with her new belief of "I now have choices," she began to take a more active role in her pelvic pain treatment. She noticed small changes in her pelvic pain and resumed treatment with the pelvic/sexual pain specialist. The hopelessness had finally shifted to a more grounded attitude of "let me see how healthy I can get."

### Joy Despite Limitations

After about six months of therapy in which we mainly focused on processing traumatic memories with EMDR therapy, we discussed new treatment goals now that the traumatic memories had been processed. Rebecca explained that she wanted increase emotional intimacy and physical intimacy with her husband, something that had drastically changed since her accident. An additional goal was to find joy and pleasure in the activities she was able to engage in. Due to the severity of Rebecca's pelvis fracture, she would never be able to return to the very active lifestyle she had before. It was also unknown if she would ever be able to have penetrative sex again. However, her other healthcare providers believed she could still make significant improvements from where she current was in terms of her lifestyle and physical activity. It was a delicate balance between being hopeful but also realistic.

Her husband Jacob attended a session to discuss the idea of improving their emotional and physical intimacy. Both agreed their relationship dynamic had changed since the accident to Jacob being a caregiver, which neither liked nor found to be conducive for sexual desire. The couple identified strategies for increasing Rebecca's independence and reducing Jacob's time in the caregiver role. Rebecca still needed Jacob to drive her everywhere due to her needing to lie down, but one of the goals she had in physical therapy was to be able to drive by herself for up to 20 minutes, allowing her to run errands and go to most of her medical appointments by herself. Rebecca's pain had decreased to a more manageable level, also allowing her to reevaluate some of the medications she was taking. She was able to reduce the dosage and even stop some of her medications that were being used to manage the chronic pain. Rebecca agreed to consult with a psychiatrist I had referred her to and to her surprise found Cymbalta seemed to slightly reduce her pain and improve her mood.

These overall medication changes afforded Rebecca more energy to engage in other activities. Rebecca was now able to stand for about 20-minute increments, and her strength continued to improve. Given this, Rebecca stated she wanted to take over cooking most of their meals, as this was something she previously had enjoyed and was mostly an achievable task now. Jacob admitted in the session feeling overwhelmed by managing all the household tasks and still working fulltime. Because the couple had the financial means to do so, we discussed what other tasks could be outsourced. The couple agreed to increase the frequency of the house cleaning service, send their laundry out to be done, and hire a dog walker for a few long walks each week. Rebecca stated she also wanted to take on more of the dog care, and although she could still not walk longer than 15 minutes, she could at least take the dog on short walks and play in the yard.

Because Rebecca had more energy, they discussed trying to engage in more shared hobbies together or going out on dates (that were still manageable for Rebecca, of course). This conversation took a very emotional and tearful turn for both, as they acknowledged needing to grieve the life they had before to embrace the new possibilities. Prior to Rebecca's accident, they had an extremely active lifestyle and imagined having a very active retirement involving international travel, skiing, hiking, scuba diving, etc. Rebecca explained wanting Jacob still to have the adventurous retirement he had always dreamed of. The two acknowledged this might mean Rebecca being "left behind" for some adventures with mutual friends and family. While Jacob was working for a few more years, Rebecca aimed for her focus to be on improving her health as much as possible to see to what extent she would be able to partake in certain adventures.

As a couple, they agreed to focus on what they could share together for the moment, which, as Rebecca put it, "Isn't much but is more than before." They acknowledged this would be a fluid situation, as sometimes treatment would flare up Rebecca's symptoms, but that at least overall her health was slowly improving. The couple identified going on short walks, eating at least one meal together daily, reading together, and watching sporting events on television as mutually enjoyable activities they wanted to start to do more of. If Rebecca's health improved, the couple both hoped to add more active and outdoor activities.

In terms of sexual intimacy, we reviewed the traditional steps of sensate focus exercises for couples. The first step of sensate focus felt too daunting to Rebecca, but the couple identified the shared goal of "just start touching again" or adding in more affection throughout their daily life. Once comfortable with affection again, the couple progressed through sensate focus exercises over the next several months. Ultimately, they became comfortable with some outercourse activities and sensual activities like taking a bath together or cuddling naked in bed.

## Siobhan

During our first session together, Siobhan admitted she was most motivated to finally address her vaginismus due to wanting to have a child naturally, not because she wanted to have penetrative sex with her husband. As a 33-year-old married Catholic woman who for religious reasons would not consider fertility treatments as a method to conceive, her time to have a child naturally was quickly dwindling. Although she had been married to her husband Tom for five years, the couple had not yet had penetrative sex. Both had waited until marriage to engage in sexual activity, so neither had much sexual experience. When they did engage in outercourse, which was rare, Siobhan kept her underwear on and was highly anxious. Tom usually left these interactions feeling frustrated and unsure of how to help his wife become more comfortable with sex.

Siobhan came from a working-class Irish Catholic family just outside of Philadelphia. She was the third of six children and had over 30 first cousins. Her father worked as an HVAC technician, and her mother worked part time as one of the secretaries for the local parish. Siobhan was a quiet and compliant child who grew up to be a quiet and compliant adult. She described her childhood as "uneventful, which is good, but it also means boring." Siobhan explained other than spending time with her family and being involved in church activities, she did not have much "fun." She did enjoy the family's yearly summer vacation for one week at the New Jersey shore. She denied experiencing trauma, including unwanted sexual experiences.

Siobhan did not receive sex education and was told at school, at church, and by her parents that sex was for marriage only. She did not self-explore and had never looked at her genitals or for that matter an image of female genitalia at all. Even in the shower, she only quickly washed her genitals with a washcloth and "really tried not to even think about it." She explained that her parents forbade dating until she was 18, which Siobhan was okay with as she was not interested in dating until young adulthood. When Siobhan was in high school, her older brother got his girlfriend pregnant while at college. "My parents basically forced them to get married. . . . I mean she wanted to, but he did not. They have a terrible marriage. My brother has never forgiven them for that, I don't think."

She attended a local Catholic university but lived at home to save money and because her parents worried about the negative influence of living with peers in a dorm. After all, as her parents pointed out, her older brother had lived away for college and ended up getting his girlfriend pregnant. She excelled as an accounting major during college and was also involved in various volunteer activities. She noticed crushes on boys during college and was pursued by a few; however, she never saw them for more than a date or two. She had only allowed one of them to kiss her. Her friends accused her of being "too picky" and often teased her about her pattern of bailing after a date or two. Siobhan explained that she was fearful of "things going further physically" and viewed her virginity as something she had to protect.

After college, Siobhan secured an entry-level accounting position and continued to live at home. Her older sister had recently married and had her first child, which made Siobhan suddenly feel pressure to get married. She attempted online dating but felt discouraged by the men she was meeting who "always seemed to want to hook-up after the first date." Siobhan met Tom at a friend's Christmas party. He, too, came from a large Catholic family and worked for his family's successful business. "We were serious from the beginning. I made it clear I was dating to get married. We get along well, and he really is my best friend," Siobhan explained during our assessment, "which also makes it more insane that I won't have sex with him. There is no one else I trust more in the world, but I still can't do it."

Like many women with lifelong vaginismus, the belief that the condition will somehow magically resolve after marriage was something Siobhan had believed. On their honeymoon, the couple kissed, but any attempt by Tom to become more physically intimate led her to experiencing panic. On the last night of the honeymoon, Siobhan recalled crying and feeling that she had failed as a woman and as a wife. Despite these strong feelings, she continued to avoid the issue. Tom, of course, colluded in his own way, immediately backing off from any touch as soon as Siobhan expressed any anxiety. The couple always wanted to have a few children, and now at 33 years old, Siobhan was faced with the reality that her issues around sexual contact were not resolving, and they were preventing her from becoming pregnant. Tom also seemed more depressed about their lack of physical intimacy and had even told her recently he was embarrassed and felt less of a man because they had not been able to achieve penetrative sex.

## Meeting Clients Where They Are

Siobhan had been diagnosed with vulvodynia by her OB/GYN after "leaping off the table" during her first attempted pelvic exam at age 30. However, given her lifelong reports of catastrophic thoughts about sex; inability to tolerate any kind of penetration, including a tampon or pelvic exam; and very phobic like responses to her own body, husband's body, and sex in general, I questioned if she had lifelong vaginismus instead. During the assessment phase of treatment,

I referred Siobhan to an OB/GYN specialist for a second opinion; the OB/GYN diagnosed her with lifelong vaginismus. The doctor was unable to assess for pelvic floor dysfunction because Siobhan's anxiety prevented her from being able to tolerate an internal exam.

"I think it would be like getting stabbed with a sword," Siobhan admitted when I asked her what she imagined penetrative sex might be like. Her imagined experience of sex was told with dread and disgust. She had a similar reaction to recounting the light outercourse she and her husband did engage in on rare occasion. She also stated she had never touched or seen her own vulva, and despite acknowledging this was strange for her age, she explained, "I really don't have a desire to see it. Ever."

In creating an exposure therapy ladder with any pelvic/sexual pain client, you must meet the client where they are. For many clients, step one is not the insertion of dilator one, and in fact, there may be several steps before a client is even ready to purchase a dilator set. Siobhan first needed to become much more comfortable with her own anatomy before entertaining the idea of dilator therapy. We first focused on psychoeducation about human anatomy and the sexual response cycle. Once Siobhan processed this new knowledge, we then shifted our focus to challenging her cognitive distortions about sex and her own body. She needed to at least come to a place where she could have a neutral reaction towards her own body and sex instead of disgust and fear. After progressing through exposure therapy using medical images, we had Siobhan engage in a set of progressive self-touch exercises, leading up to looking at her own genitals in a hand mirror. This phase of the therapeutic work took about six months.

The next steps were for Siobhan to order the dilators and simply get used to having them around. Initially, the dilators felt very scary and threatening to Siobhan. "I can't even imagine putting that thing anywhere near my body," she explained. I instructed her to spend some time with dilator number one while doing activities around her home like cooking, watching television, reading a book, etc. Once her anxiety decreased, we then had her touch the dilator to her arms and legs but not near her genital area. Next, we had her touch dilator number one to her genitals with her underwear on. However, it was the following step that Siobhan felt completely paralyzed by. In fact, Siobhan rated her anxiety about touching the dilator to her genitals without underwear on (even without any insertion) an 8 of 10 on the anxiety scale.

We discussed using EMDR therapy as an option for Siobhan to overcome her phobic anxiety regarding penetration. EMDR therapy can serve as a form of exposure therapy when working with a "future template" or imagining a future event. During EMDR therapy, Siobhan imaged herself confronting her anxiety about touching dilator number one to her genital area (or nesting the dilator). The EMDR session provided her the space to imagine successfully overcoming her phobic anxiety and completing the exposure therapy step. Siobhan returned to session the following week radiating with confidence and proclaimed that she had been able to touch the dilator to her genital area. Siobhan requested to do EMDR therapy for the next several exposure therapy steps to help her achieve penetration with dilator number one. After two months of rehearsing each step with EMDR therapy, she was able to insert dilator number one. To her pleasant surprise, there was not pain, and she was able to manage her anxiety successfully. She made slow and steady progress the following six months moving through the other dilators but did not request EMDR therapy for these additional steps. After nearly a year of psychotherapy and working with an OB/GYN specialist, Siobhan was ready to transition to penetrative sex.

### Boundaries

Homework related to moving through the exposure therapy ladder always requires time. Many clients struggle with setting aside the time for physical therapy, stretching, or doing dilators for legitimate reasons like lack of childcare, being overworked, experiencing burnout, caretaking for a parent, etc. However, it is important for therapists who work with clients who have pelvic/sexual pain to be on the lookout for those who use other activities or demands as avoidance. Early in therapy, it became clear Siobhan was avoiding or at least putting dilator therapy last on her list of priorities.

"Tom said he doesn't believe I want kids because I'm not taking the time to do the things that will get us there [i.e., dilators]," Siobhan said tearfully about four months into treatment. He had a point. Siobhan had become the default babysitter for her older sister's three children, often spending multiple nights a week and even a weekend day watching them. And often if Siobhan was the default babysitter, this meant Tom was as well. According to Siobhan, he was reaching a "breaking point" about the situation. She admitted that her sister often "dumps them without even giving notice" and that "Tom doesn't believe I'm actually upset about it because I don't tell her to stop." The additional childcare Siobhan was doing for her sister's children consumed most of her free time, meaning dilator therapy and the couple's sensate focus exercises rarely happened. "Tom says we're going to lose our chance to have children because I'm too busy taking care of my sisters'," Siobhan reported.

Siobhan had a long history of struggling to set boundaries with others, including her family. The family expectation was to "help each other" regardless of the personal consequences. She had grown up watching her parents give away money they did not have to help extended family. At one point, her aunt and cousins lived with them for a year in their already overcrowded house. One of her older cousin's was struggling with opiate addiction and had stolen from their family. She recalled feeling very unsafe around him. Once when she was sick and home from school, he invited a stranger into their house, who she assumed was a drug dealer. All the adults were at work. Siobhan remembered trying to pretend like she was asleep as the stranger noticed her alone in her bedroom. A brief window of opportunity presented itself, and she ran down the hall and locked herself in the bathroom, which she stayed in for the next several hours until her mother came home.

"Nothing happened to me, so I don't consider it sexual trauma. I don't know what to call it. I told my mom when she got home, but my cousin denied anyone even being in the house," Siobhan stated. Although an extreme example, it did highlight her feeling of not being protected by her family or that her own needs did not matter. It was the identical message she was hearing from her mom now as an adult. "I tried to explain, you know without giving private details, that I needed more time to take care of some things for myself and did not want to babysit anymore. And all my mom said was, 'What about your sister? She can't go to work if she doesn't have childcare.'" Attempting to set a boundary with her sister went equally as poor. Her sister lashed out at her, accusing Tom and her of being selfish for not helping, asking, "Don't you want to spend time with your nieces and nephews?"

After agreeing to watch her nieces and nephew one night a week instead of multiple nights, her sister continued to violate this boundary by dropping them off for unscheduled visits. This behavior put Siobhan and Tom in a difficult situation. They knew they risked alienation from her family if they enforced the boundary, but without the boundary enforcement, they risked further deterioration of their marriage. I referred Siobhan and Tom to a couple's therapist, where they would have the space to process this difficult decision as a couple. Meanwhile, in individual therapy, we processed Siobhan's feelings about her needs not mattering while growing up and how as an adult she often allowed others to treat her in this way.

Our work shifted to learning assertive communication skills and healthy boundary setting, which she first began to implement at work. For Siobhan, work felt like a safer place to experiment with assertiveness skills and boundary setting rather than with her family. She was well liked by her supervisors at her accounting firm and was known as a very hard worker. One of her coworkers, however, tended to take credit for her work on some large client accounts they shared. And while it had always bothered her, she had avoided confronting him and was fearful to "cause an issue." After practicing assertiveness skills in session and at places like the grocery store or at a doctor's appointment, Siobhan gained enough confidence to confront her coworker. And while he disagreed with her perception of the situation, she felt proud for confronting him and later decided to disclose the issue to her direct supervisor, which resulted in her being paired with a different coworker who was a better fit for her work style.

Concurrently, her couples therapy work had helped Tom and her come to decide to confront her parents and sister about using them for childcare. Because her sister had already disregarded the boundary they previously attempted to set and because the couple now recognized the amount of time needed to work towards achieving penetrative sex, they decided to set a firm boundary that they were no longer available to help with any childcare. As expected, and luckily prepared for thanks to the work they had done in couples' therapy, Siobhan's sister and parents reacted very angrily and unsupportively. However, the experience had united the couple and made them feel as though they were working towards the goal of penetrative sex more collaboratively.

## Noemi

When Noemi entered therapy, she was experiencing a range of PTSD symptoms, but she had been misdiagnosed by her OB/GYN as having postpartum depression. Many clinicians and doctors may confuse the symptoms of PTSD with postpartum depression. While there may be some overlap in symptoms such as having difficulty bonding with the baby, feeling sad or having a low mood, losing interest in activities once enjoyed, difficulty sleeping, and withdrawing socially, the importance between these two disorders is significant. In addition, the course of treatment between postpartum depression versus PTSD is different, and therefore obtaining a correct diagnosis is crucial.

In Noemi's case, the qualifying event for a PTSD diagnosis was the postpartum hemorrhage in which she nearly lost her life. She experienced intrusive memories about the event and avoided people, places, and things that reminded her of the hemorrhage, including sometimes her own daughter and stepson. She felt extremely ashamed of this and was relieved to hear that PTSD might explain this reaction. When Noemi felt triggered by the trauma, she would experience anxiety or panic and often become very irritable. She also continued to feel that she was to blame for the hemorrhage and that if she had "only pushed harder for the doctors to listen to me," that it could have been avoided. The blame she placed on herself was very exaggerated, another sign of PTSD. Noemi also reported being extremely distressed by the memories of her sexual assault coming up since her medical trauma.

Noemi grew up in a working-class neighborhood just outside of Philadelphia. Her father was a first-generation immigrant from a Latin American country, and her mother was a second-generation Italian American. Her father owned a contracting business, and her mother worked as a nurse. She described her family as warm, fun, and "very emotionally expressive." She was the middle child and had an older brother and a younger sister. Noemi reported being raised Catholic, and although she only identified as a "major holiday Catholic," for her parents, their religion was extremely important. She grew up very close to both sides of her extended family and spent a few weeks every summer visiting with her father's sister and cousins abroad. Both parents placed value on education, especially her father, who viewed anything less than an A as unacceptable. Noemi did well in school and excelled in running cross country and track, for which she later received a scholarship to a large state school. Noemi did date in college but "never anything seriously" and denied any traumatic events, including unwanted sexual experiences, until her assault at work.

"My father was so proud of the job I landed out of college. It killed me to have to leave the position. He is still upset about it, I think." Noemi had left her job after being sexually assaulted by a senior member of the company. She never disclosed the sexual assault to her family due to feeling like she might be to blame in some way and that it would also "kill my father." She luckily found another company that she enjoyed working for after a few transitional jobs. She met her husband Nick through friends in her late 20s. "He was different than the other guys I had met. He had a quiet seriousness about him that I liked. He had a son and ran his own business – he was a man," she explained about what drew her to Nick. Noemi stated it took a while for her father to approve of Nick since he had a child outside of marriage, "but my father eventually said that at least he was doing the right thing by raising his son." Noemi was hesitant about dating Nick at first due to his having a child and him being the primary caregiver. The mother struggled with addiction, had lost most of her custody, and was rarely around. "This meant if I was going to be with Nick long term, I had to get on board with being a mom, too. Nick always said that they were a 'two-package deal.'"

They got married after dating for two years and immediately started trying for a child of their own. They struggled with infertility, but with some medical intervention, Noemi was able to become pregnant. She was elated, yet the timing was distressing due to news leaking about her former company covering up reports of sexual assaults for years. "I remember when my father saw it on the news, he asked me about it. Flat out asked if that is what happened to me, you know, because of how abruptly I had left before. I told him no, but I can tell he doesn't believe me. But I was pregnant and just didn't want to deal with any more stress." Noemi, of course, did end up having to deal with a lot more stress after nearly losing her life a few days after the birth of her daughter from a postpartum hemorrhage. In saving her life, the doctors needed to perform an emergency hysterectomy. Due to all the trauma symptoms she was experiencing, she had not yet been able to process the grief around this loss.

Our immediate treatment focus was to reduce the PTSD symptoms by processing both the sexual assault and the medical trauma using EMDR therapy. "Why are these memories linked up for me? How is a sexual assault like the medical trauma?" Noemi initially wondered. Through EMDR therapy, however, we realized that both traumatic events had left her with the same feeling – not being in control or being powerless. Initially Noemi felt pressure to resolve her pelvic/sexual pain because she believed her marriage was in a fragile state. I encouraged her to prioritize treating the PTSD symptoms first, as trauma can sometimes become a barrier when trying to treat pelvic/sexual pain. However, Noemi insisted on trying to start pelvic floor physical therapy. We discussed the pros and cons of her starting physical therapy before processing her trauma and ultimately Noemi still decided to try physical therapy.

### When the Treatment of Pelvic/Sexual Pain is a Trigger

"It was too much," Noemi admitted as if she thought she were in trouble during our session after she had started pelvic floor physical therapy. I reassured her that it was okay for her to try pelvic floor physical therapy, and we reframed the experience as her developing a better understanding of where she is in terms of the therapeutic work. Common treatments for clients with pelvic/sexual pain often include pelvic floor physical therapy, dilator therapy, receiving injections, or using suppositories. These treatments can be extremely triggering for those with medical or sexual trauma, and it is common for these past traumas to get reactivated while a woman is undergoing these treatments.

In addition, all these treatments require time, energy, and financial resources. Undergoing counseling for trauma also requires the same resources. These resources do not exist in an infinite amount, and clients often must make difficult choices about what to treat first. In my experience, if a client is living with PTSD symptoms, trauma must be treated first. If the traumatic experiences are not interfering with the client's day-to-day functioning, pelvic/sexual pain could be treated first; however, both the clinician and the client should look for signs that treatment is becoming too triggering. Signs that trauma needs to be treated first include:

1. *Experiencing intrusive memories about the trauma:* Clients who begin to experience intrusive memories about their trauma after starting the physical treatment of their pelvic/sexual pain often need counseling. Noemi reported feeling very panicked by the prospect of an internal physical exam by the physical therapist and experienced distressing memories about her sexual assault. Clients who attempt to push through these triggers will often find themselves starting to avoid treatment and experiencing an increase of their pelvic/sexual pain–related symptoms.

2. *Sleep disruptions:* Noemi stated she was having trouble staying asleep and sometimes had distressing nightmares about both traumatic events. In discussing both physical and emotional healing in treatment, we talked about the importance of quality sleep. Clients experiencing significant sleep disruptions due to PTSD symptoms will be too emotionally and physically drained to get the most out of treatment.

3. *Lack of progress:* Clients who do not address traumatic experiences that interfere with pelvic/sexual pain treatment may find themselves not making the progress they had hoped. There may be a general sense of feeling stuck, and both the client and the healthcare provider may feel puzzled by the lack of progress.

4. *An increase in anxiety and/or depression symptoms:* After Noemi's appointment with the pelvic/floor physical therapist. she noted an increase of her anxiety symptoms. Clients who notice this increase in anxiety and depression symptoms may need to address any traumatic experiences that could be getting stirred up.

5. *Dissociation:* Sometimes clients who have traumatic experiences may dissociate or numb out during the physical treatment of pelvic/sexual pain. Sadly, dissociation can often be confused with quiet compliance. Any dissociation during treatment could be a red flag that trauma may need to be addressed.

6. *Guarding or clenching:* Noemi noted that she found herself clenching her pelvic floor muscles once in the exam room with the pelvic

floor physical therapist. Any guarding or clenching will make progress with pelvic floor physical therapy or dilator therapy extremely difficult.

Once Noemi understood the importance of first addressing her trauma, she agreed to trying EDMR therapy. Because Noemi was anxious about the state of her marriage and the lack of physical affection, we asked Noemi's husband to attend a session to discuss what the couple could work on until Noemi was both emotionally and physically ready to start working on rebuilding their sexual intimacy. With an explanation of the treatment process, Noemi's husband was onboard with the temporary break from penetrative sex and certain outercourse activities. Noemi and her husband agreed to focus on reconnecting with nondemand touch such as cuddling, kissing, exchanging massage, etc. They also agreed to implement a date night that each of them would take turns planning.

### Reclaiming the Body

Once Noemi's trauma symptoms were significantly reduced after EMDR therapy, grief started to set in. There were many layers to her grief, including grief over the consequences of her sexual assault and consequences of her postpartum hemorrhage. "I think before, I was just happy to be alive and was living moment to moment under the stress of having a newborn. I didn't really have a chance to process the hysterectomy, let alone the other body changes from pregnancy and motherhood," Noemi reflected one session. This felt like her experience after the sexual assault when the crisis of leaving her job and finding a new job demanded her focus rather than the actual trauma that had occurred. In both situations, she was never able to pause and process the gravity of what had happened to her or her body.

Noemi's self-proclaimed strategy of "tucking it away" only worked mentally. She realized through therapy that her body had always remembered and was holding on to the trauma. It was in the work of attempting to transition back to penetrative sex that unveiled the complicated emotions she held towards her body. She was angry at her body in almost a victim-blaming kind of way for making her a target for a sexual assault. The postpartum hemorrhage and resulting hysterectomy also made her feel "let down" by her body. Noemi also admitted struggling with liking her postpartum body and was also experiencing the normal feeling of being "touched out."

After EMDR therapy, Noemi had begun pelvic floor physical therapy. After about six months of pelvic floor physical therapy and dilator therapy, her physical therapist felt she was physically ready to attempt penetrative sex. Emotionally, Noemi was not ready. "I feel like I should feel proud that I made all this progress, but honestly, I kind of just feel full of dread. I want to want to have sex so Nick can be happier, but I don't really see the point of it for me," she lamented. Noemi's low sexual desire seemed driven by normal postpartum feelings and the negative emotions Noemi was experiencing about her body.

Our work shifted to focusing on how Noemi could both reclaim her body and be comfortable with her new sexual self. I suspected if she could accomplish these two things the sexual desire issue would resolve. Together we identified the following strategies Noemi would try:

1. *Develop a more positive body image:* Because Noemi felt poorly about her body, she avoided physical contact with Nick and being naked around him. This obviously reduced opportunities for them to connect sexually. Noemi began to create a list of the things she appreciated about her body, which included both practical functioning and what she called "my sex appeal." She kept this list on her phone so it was easily accessible and would refer to the list when she was experiencing negative thoughts about her body.

2. *Get more sleep:* Noemi realized her lack of sleep was negatively impacting her mood and robbing her of energy to engage with Nick even in non-sexual ways. After consulting with her pediatrician, Noemi decided to stop breastfeeding in the hopes of being able to get more sleep. She also decided to try her best to nap once a day while her daughter was napping (instead of spending this time rushing around doing chores). After a few weeks of having made these changes, Noemi did notice improvements in her mood and energy level. She also found it easier to challenge the negative stories she told herself about her body, which she attributed to more sleep.

3. *Move:* Noemi had identified her years competing as a runner during college as a time when she had a very positive attitude towards her body. Of course, she looked healthy and fit while running as a college athlete, but she explained she got more out of feeling connected to her body and being able to feel like she accomplished something with her body whether it was completing a workout or winning a race. Noemi began a progressive walk-to-run program designed by her pelvic floor physical therapist. She began to look forward to this time, as it was a form of self-care and made her feel good about what her body was still capable of despite all the trauma she had been through. "I think out of all of the changes I made, working up to running again and making that commitment to myself has been the biggest help in shifting my attitude towards my body. Yeah, it's been through some bad shit, but it's still capable of amazing things," she later told me. Noemi also joined a local running club, which helped reduced her social isolation as a new mom.

4. *Schedule time to physically connect:* Noemi decided to confront her avoidance of intimacy more directly by scheduling two 30-minute times during the week to connect physically with Nick. While the intention was to engage in something more sexual (like outercourse until she was emotionally ready for penetrative sex), cuddling, taking a bath or shower together, or doing massage together was also okay. The focus was for the experiences to be non-demand touch and mutually pleasurable. Scheduling allowed Noemi to identify the most ideal times for her during the week when she could consider factors like sleep and stress. Through scheduling, Noemi realized that generally earlier in the day was better for her, and she also began to find herself looking forward to these times with Nick.

5. *Increase " foreplay" throughout the day:* "Foreplay" starts from the moment you wake up! This includes light touching, flirty texts throughout the day, a simple "how's your day going" check-in, sharing tasks at home, etc. Sometimes couples neglect these small but important interactions, which decrease opportunities for women to experience the type of foreplay they need to be open to the possibility of sex later. Both Nick and Noemi agreed to make a concerted effort engaging with each other in this way. They later noticed how this

helped them to feel more connected throughout the day and feel more positive about their relationship.

6.   *Outsource:* The reality was that for Noemi to be able to run, get more sleep, find time to physically connect with Nick, and make time for pelvic floor physical therapy, she needed time. While we cannot add more hours to the day, we can outsource tasks or get more help. To essentially "buy back time," the couple agreed to begin ordering groceries and pharmacy items online to be delivered. They picked a healthy meal kit to be delivered two days a week, saving them some time with cooking. Through this experience, Nick also realized he needed to take on more of the household management. The couple also agreed to accept more help from Nick's mother and Noemi's younger sister, who wanted to be more involved with their children's lives. They also made changes in their budget so that they could have cleaners for their home twice a month.

## Important Takeaways

- Despite our fragmented healthcare systems and unique barriers that each client faces, pelvic/sexual pain disorders and sexual trauma can still be treated concurrently and successfully.
- Each client will have a different starting point in psychotherapy, but effective treatment will always depend on the integration of a multimodal approach, including collaboration with other healthcare provider and using evidenced-based treatments.
- Acknowledging barriers such as financial limitations, lack of time, limited insurance coverage for the treatment of pelvic/sexual pain, and other life demands ground treatment in the realities our clients face.

# 9

## CASE VIGNETTES – TERMINATION

DOI: 10.4324/9781003168232-9

## Ideal and Not-so-Ideal Conditions for Termination

Termination for each of the case vignettes will be reviewed in this chapter, highlighting some of the normal but less than ideal conditions that can lead to termination. Under ideal conditions, treatment termination is guided by reaching the collaborative goals established by the client and the therapist. Once these goals are accomplished, a relapse prevention plan should be created, and treatment can be terminated. When working with clients who have pelvic/sexual pain, there are a few general indicators that termination may be appropriate. First, the client has received appropriate medical care and has an effective treatment team established. For those for whom penetrative sex was not a treatment goal, the client has been able to reach whatever goal around penetration they identified as being important such as inserting a tampon without pain or being able to tolerate a pelvic exam. For clients who had a treatment goal of achieving penetrative sex, the client should be able to achieve pain-free intercourse upon termination. If the client will always have some level of pain due to their medical conditions, the client has strategies to work around the pain such as knowing the ideal conditions for making penetrative sex most comfortable and enjoyable and having a broad sexual menu that includes many non-penetrative activities.

Other signs that a client is ready to terminate include being able to communicate with a partner about their sexual/pelvic pain symptoms and the ability to initiate non-penetrative sensual or sexual activities are still enjoyable if they are experiencing a flare-up of symptoms. Generally, clients should leave therapy having a varied and broad sexual menu, and if they are partnered, the couple should already feel confident navigating around the pelvic/sexual pain. Clients should demonstrate effective communication skills to use with partners and their treatment teams. Clients with traumatic pasts will have processed their traumatic experiences and experience significantly less posttraumatic stress disorder (PTSD)–like symptoms and experiences of "feeling triggered." Grief and anger around "what could have been" without having experienced a traumatic event and/or pelvic/sexual pain disorder will be processed, and clients will have coping skills for confronting these complex emotions when they arise in the future. Clients will have developed effective anxiety and/or depression coping skills and chronic pain management techniques.

As we know, circumstances are not always ideal. Termination occurs due to a client's life changes such as relocating, experiencing a significant financial hardship, or experiencing another crisis that takes priority over their treatment. Sometimes changes in the therapist's life might make treatment no longer possible. There are a few common themes I have seen play out with clients who have pelvic/sexual pain disorders when termination occurs under less-than-ideal circumstances:

1.    *Time commitment conflicts:* It takes significant time and energy to address a pelvic/sexual pain disorder. Clients often must juggle appointments with multiple providers, as well as their work and family obligations. They must also carve out time at home to do dilator therapy, stretching, or other physical therapy exercises. If clients are struggling with how to balance treatment with their other commitments, first try to identify with the client what the most important component of the treatment is at that moment in time. Then discuss with them how they can prioritize this one aspect of the treatment for now. Even with narrowing treatment prioritizes to one task, being able to engage in one treatment task will still means sacrificing time spent with family, work, hobbies, etc. Not everyone wants to or is able to make these changes. Overall time designated for the treatment of the pelvic/sexual pain disorder could also be reduced, but it is important to communicate with the client that this will slow progress. If clients cannot set aside time to practice dilators for 15 minutes two times a week, try a new anxiety-coping skill, attend a monthly appointment with a specialist, etc., then progress is highly unlikely. It is important to normalize for these clients that if they are unable to carve out some time towards treatment, it is okay to put treatment on hold. I try to reframe the process around this decision as their still deciding how they want to approach treatment for their pelvic/sexual pain disorder. I also reassure them that now that they understand the treatment process, they can work towards making changes in their schedules so they can reengage in the treatment process.

2.    *Yearning for a magical solution:* Occasionally, I see a client who despite understanding the treatment process will continue to fixate on wanting a magical solution. These clients usually do not commit much time to treatment, even if they have the time. And despite not engaging in the treatment recommendations, at each appointment, they express shock and disappointment. Those looking for a quick fix are also more likely to dismiss their gains when they do make improvements. Because they are so focused on their long-term goal not happening overnight, they seem to ignore the small steps forward. For some, this presentation could be a result of depression, which should then take the precedent in treatment. For others, however, their desire for a magical cure that will never arrive may be related to secondary gain issues that we may never be made privy to. Some clients looking for a magical solution may tell you they are unwilling to engage in any of the treatment options available to them, sometimes known as the "yeah, but . . ." group of clients. Even when presented with evidenced-based treatments and the length of time these treatments typically require before seeing improvements, they request other options. I gently explain that these are the treatment approaches we know work and that I do not have any other tools in my toolbox, so to speak. With clients yearning for a magical solution, I often have a direct conversation about expectations versus reality and what can be gained from treatment versus what cannot be. We also discuss my role as a therapist and the types of treatment I can offer versus what I cannot offer. For some, this conversation can become a turning point in the therapeutic process, while others decide to terminate.

3.    *Wanting partnered sex to not be an option:* Sometimes during therapy, clients with pelvic/sexual pain disorders come to realize they do not want to have penetrative sex with their partner, even if they are able to physically get to a place where they could. For clients coming from extremely religious or conservative backgrounds, there may be a sexual orientation conflict they are unwilling to acknowledge or face due to cultural norms. Others have admitted to me that having a pelvic/sexual pain disorder and thus being unable to have penetrative sex was essentially the only form of birth control

available to them and that they did not want to have any more children. Another woman from a strict religious background admitted in treatment that she believed her husband was having an affair, and having a medical reason not to engage in penetrative sex was the only way to keep herself sexually safe because divorce was not sanctioned by her religion. Reasons that women in heterosexual relationships commonly cite for no longer wanting to have sex with their partners include not feeling supported by their partners, feeling resentful by the additional tasks they take on at home and with children, or realizing there is abuse going on in the relationship. When this happens, it is possible to reassess and create new goals that do not involve partner penetration, like, for instance, only working up to dilator number two or three, which would allow for toleration of a pelvic exam. The goals can also focus more on quality-of-life issues rather than emotional or physical intimacy with the partner. Some women will still decide to leave therapy, and I have had some women explicitly tell me that their decision is mostly driven by not wanting their partner to think they will be able to have penetrative sex again.

4.   *Substance abuse issues:* Due to years of untreated chronic pain, some women with pelvic/sexual pain disorders have turned to self-medicating with alcohol or drugs. Other women have been prescribed opiates by their physicians and become addicted. On rare occasion, I have worked with a pelvic/sexual pain client who could not even stay awake during the first session due to suspected alcohol or opiate abuse. It is not appropriate to continue working with clients who are unable to engage in treatment due to drug or alcohol abuse. In these situations, I encourage clients to discuss their medication regimen with the prescribing doctor before continuing therapy. I require that I be able to speak to the prescribing physician, of which many clients whom I suspect are abusing their medications, refuse. When appropriate, I make a referral to a drug or alcohol program or specialist. Some clients may take this referral, while others, especially those being prescribed opiates by a physician, may become irate by the suggestion they may have to address their pain medication dependence. Regardless of the reaction, termination is appropriate in these situations.

## Termination in the Case Vignettes

### *Paula*

Due to Paula's moving to another state for graduate school, therapy was terminated prior to her meeting all her therapeutic goals. However, once Paula knew she would be relocating by the spring of her senior year of college, we spent a considerable amount of time connecting her to a new treatment team. Luckily, Paula was moving to a large West Coast city, where she was able to find a pelvic floor physical therapist and an OB/GYN who specialized in pelvic/sexual pain disorders. Finding a psychotherapist who was familiar with pelvic/sexual pain proved more difficult. However, because of the gains she made in treatment for her pelvic/sexual pain disorder, she decided to focus on finding a psychotherapist who specialized in trauma and obsessive-compulsive disorder.

Paula had made significant progress during treatment. Most of her posttraumatic stress disorder (PTSD)–symptoms had subsided, and she had developed effective coping skills to manage her anxiety. She was also communicating more assertively with others in her life. Through pelvic floor physical therapy and medication, she experienced significant improvement with her pelvic/sexual pain symptoms. She was able to have penetrative sex without pain 75% of the time and was able to wear tampons comfortably. Her boyfriend from college would be relocating with her, and both were excited to take the next step of living together. Both Paula and her boyfriend were motivated in continuing to make penetrative sex more comfortable. They had broadened their sexual menu and felt confident in adding more outercourse activities when penetrative sex was not possible. At the end of therapy, Paula noted how the experience of pelvic/sexual pain forced her and her boyfriend to know themselves better sexually and to develop a deeper connection. "Between supporting me through the trial and pelvic pain stuff, I know we're able to get through difficult things together, and it says a lot about who he is as a person and who we are as a couple," Paula noted during one of our last sessions.

We spent time discussing where Paula wanted her therapeutic work to go moving forward with her new therapist. Paula acknowledged she was struggling more recently with grief, especially around how her college experience would have been different if she were not going through a trial and dealing with PTSD symptoms most of the time. She had tried to separate herself from her family's decision to move, but she emotionally felt it was her "fault." It did not, of course, help that her youngest sister's high school experience had been disrupted by the move and she was openly angry towards Paula. Her parents also overshared their own emotional experiences about what had happened to Paula, which she found distressing. Knowing how much her parents were torturing themselves over having not been able to protect Paula made her feel guilty and like she needed to protect them. She identified needing to maintain healthy boundaries with her family as one of her new therapy goals.

Going through the trial while also treating her pelvic/sexual pain highlighted the mind–body connection for Paula. Using the pain and anxiety scales showed her that high stress or anxiety usually flared her symptoms. Entering graduate school, Paula knew she would need to work on stress management for both her mental and pelvic/sexual pain. We identified other campus and community resources Paula could connect with if she found herself struggling with stress management. And although we could certainly not predict her graduate school schedule, we reviewed the time management techniques and stress reduction skills that had helped her during college.

Another important goal for Paula was to have an academic experience that was "not so tied up in my trauma and the trial." Paula's graduate program would be two years, coincidentally, the same amount of time her perpetrator had been given probation. Like many of my clients whose sexual assault cases enter the justice system, Paula left feeling disappointed and angry. "I'm afraid I'll keep making these mental comparisons throughout my program. The closer I get to finishing my master's degree, the closer he gets to being done with his already short sentence," Paula explained. We identified other possible trauma triggers, and Paula agreed sign a release of information for her new psychotherapist so I would be able to inform her about the legal saga and resulting angst.

## Violet

After about a year of treatment, Violet felt more secure in her long-term treatment plan and believed her symptoms were being managed well. She would always have some degree of pain and other autoimmune-like symptoms due to the endometriosis but reported having a better understanding of the disease and how to navigate her flareups. She continued with a home-based physical therapy program and acupuncture twice a month. Violet stated that she wanted to continue with "monthly check-ins" with me while she made the transition out of teaching as she anticipated this being a stressful time. During these sessions, we explored options for her that would afford greater financial stability and provide a work–life balance that would enable her to focus on her health. The process of searching for a new career was triggering for Violet and stirred up old feelings of not knowing herself or trusting her judgement. She was putting a lot of pressure on herself to make the next career move the final career move. We spent significant time reframing the next career move as just that – a career move. Perhaps it would be something she would love and stay in long term, or perhaps it would be a more transitional step for her.

An interesting opportunity presented itself for Violet as she was contemplating her next steps. A good friend from childhood had recently bought her family's insurance business and actively recruited Violet to work for her as the business administrator for a very reasonable salary. There was also potential for Violet to become a licensed insurance agent and earn additional income. The position would require her to move back to Tennessee, which she was not opposed to due to being closer to her family and a more affordable cost of living. She would also be very close to a major city, which appealed to her. Her biggest fear, however, was reestablishing a treatment team, which felt extremely daunting given how long it took her to find her current team.

I encouraged Violet to research healthcare providers in the area so we could assess the resources for her. I also reached out to healthcare providers I knew and requested referrals for endometriosis specialists and pelvic pain specialists in the area Violet was considering moving. I received one name for a pelvic floor physical therapist in the area who Violet reached out to. Luckily, the pelvic floor physical therapist was able to provide her with other names of therapists in the community who treated clients with endometriosis and pelvic/sexual pain. Violet decided to take some days off to return home, learn more about the job, explore her possible new community, and meet with the pelvic floor physical therapist she had connected with. When she returned, she explained, "My gut is telling me to take the job and make the move, and I think I should trust my gut on this one."

After years of not trusting her gut, Violet finally did. We prepared to terminate therapy when Violet confirmed her moving date. In that time (about six weeks), we focused on her making other connections in the community such as an OB/GYN and acupuncturist. Violet reported that she did not believe she needed a psychotherapist at the time but identified an increase in her anxiety symptoms and intense feelings of self-doubt as possible signs for needing to seek counseling again. In our final sessions, we also identified how Violet could establish a healthy and happy life in her new community and home.

### Rebecca

After two years of working together, Rebecca and I discussed whether termination was appropriate. She had processed her past traumas with eye movement desensitization and reprocessing (EMDR) and was slowly but steadily improving her overall physical health, including her pelvic pain. She reported that she would continue working with her pelvic floor physical therapist, the OB/GYN specialist, and her psychiatrist. Rebecca had also added acupuncture to her treatment towards the end of our work together and intended to continue weekly treatments as she found it helped reduce her chronic pain.

Rebecca was anxious to terminate, explaining, "Things are okay now, but what if they get bad again?" Rebecca decided to reduce her appointments to "monthly check-ins" after learning she could always increase her session frequency if needed. After five "monthly check-ins" when we mainly focused on chronic pain management strategies and anxiety coping skills and identifying new activities to enjoy by herself or with her husband as her health improved, Rebecca stated she was ready to terminate therapy. Rebecca and I discussed what she wanted to continue working on even though our sessions would be ending. She acknowledged needing to continue working on challenging her cognitive distortions around her health and quality of life, especially during flare-ups of symptoms. She also wanted to continue to expand her activities as her health allowed – both in general and sexually – and "make sure I don't put myself in a prison."

Rebecca explained she was not sure if achieving penetrative sex should be a long-term goal she worked on. I was curious when she brought this up. This had been discussed between her husband and her in one of our sessions, and he stated he wanted to connect sexually with her but was okay if penetrative sex could not occur. In addition, all her healthcare providers had been clear in telling the couple that they were unsure if Rebecca would ever be able to have pain-free penetrative sex. Rebecca explained that although her husband was not pressuring her for penetrative sex, she found herself wondering if there was an unspoken hope that this could one day happen again.

We discussed, as she had been able to do with other activities, how to stay in the moment and find the joy in what she is able to do at that time. We also explored the social pressures and sexual myths regarding penetrative sex. Rebecca was able to acknowledge that her own marriage was an example counter to the social pressures and myths, showing her that penetrative sex was not necessary to have a healthy marriage. She identified the emotional and physical intimacy as "the glue that keeps us together" and that it was okay if penetrative sex was not a part of their physical intimacy. Rebecca said she wanted to "hold the hope [of penetrative sex] but not let it take away from what I can do right now."

### Siobhan

Siobhan had made significant progress during treatment, having gone from a very high phobic anxiety response towards the thought of sexual contact to being able to engage in outercourse activities that she found pleasurable. Once Siobhan was physically and emotionally ready to transition to penetrative sex, we invited her husband Tom in for a session to review the process. Before any attempt, Siobhan would pre-dilate and do diaphragmatic breathing for relaxation. The first step for the couple would be for Tom to "park the car" or simply insert without thrusting. Once the couple did this a few times without Siobhan's anxiety above a 4 of 10, they could then add a few thrusts. We invited Tom in for another session after this step was achieved to improve sexual communication skills and provide psychoeducation around sexually pleasurable activities for both. We also discussed realistic expectations for this next phase of treatment. I explained that the transition to penetrative sex would likely feel clinical and not very sensual for a while. I reassured them that once they became acquainted with the logistics of penetrative sex and Siobhan was able to engage confidently knowing she was not experiencing painful intercourse, then they would be able to focus on making the experience more sensual and pleasurable.

It took about six months for the couple to go from "parking the car" to what they called "normal sex." Siobhan stated she felt relieved and happy that penetrative sex was now a part of their marriage and that it did not involve pain. At this point, Siobhan and I both thought it was appropriate to terminate therapy. Siobhan identified wanting to continue to work on healthy boundaries and assertive communication even after therapy was terminated. Although she had made significant gains in both setting health boundaries and engaging in assertive communication, these were new skills, and she knew they needed continued practice. In addition, her family continued to disregard her boundaries, causing both personal and marriage distress. Her older sister had "basically launched a full-fledged war against me and Tom," since Siobhan and Tom explained they would no longer be helping with childcare. Having previously always been close to her family, even if it was somewhat "unhealthy enmeshment" as she now described it, Siobhan was distraught by the alienation her sister was causing.

Siobhan and Tom would continue with couples counseling to cope with continued stress related to her family and to decide about whether to pursue fertility treatment. Tom wanted them to proceed with fertility treatment, but Siobhan was nervous that this was against their religion and that her family would not accept a child born from medical intervention. However, just before termination of therapy, Siobhan's cousin had discreetly disclosed to her that she had gotten pregnant from fertility treatment. Her cousin explained they would never tell most members of the family due to the strict Catholic beliefs, but the disclosure seemed to soften Siobhan to the possibility of trying medical intervention. Before termination, we spent a few sessions processing Siobhan's conflicting beliefs and emotions around fertility treatment and fears of further alienation from her family if the couple had a child via medical intervention.

## *Noemi*

"I'll know I am ready to terminate therapy when I can feel okay having sex again – both physically and emotionally," Noemi explained when we were discussing how she would know she was ready to terminate therapy. While this statement may seem simple, there were multiple barriers Noemi had to overcome to become physically and emotionally well enough to enjoy sex again. First, she had to process the traumatic events that were interfering not only with her ability to engage in sex but also with her daily functioning. Noemi experienced significant improvements in reducing her PTSD symptoms after targeting the postpartum hemorrhage and sexual assault with EMDR therapy.

The work then shifted to treating her pelvic/sexual pain, grief, and sexual self-esteem. With a combination of at home dilator therapy and pelvic floor physical therapy, Noemi was able to reach her goal of being physically ready to have penetrative sex. However, becoming emotionally ready to engage in penetrative sex took more time. We next spent significant time processing the grief that had come up around the losses associated with the sexual assault, the pregnancy, the postpartum hemorrhage, and the hysterectomy. Noemi made several lifestyle changes that enabled her to engage in more self-care and allowed her to feel more confident and connected to her postpartum and post-hysterectomy body.

Two years after nearly dying from the postpartum hemorrhage Noemi competed in her first running race since her days as a college athlete. "Running is now a celebration of what my body is still capable of despite everything I've been through. I can still do amazing things, be healthy, and be happy with my body," she explained after completing a half-marathon. Nick's "stepping up" for her to train for the race also helped her to feel more connected to him again. It was also in training that Noemi was able to accept and embrace her new body, which resulted in her becoming more open to engaging in sexual activity with Nick again. We began to space out our sessions from every other week to a monthly check-in. Noemi felt comfortable terminating therapy a few months after the couple had resumed penetrative sex and had established a "new normal." For the couple, this new normal included carving out intentional time in their schedules to be physically intimate, trying to connect during the mornings or daytime, and engaging in more outercourse.

## My Hopes for Clinicians After Reading this Book

After reading this book, one of my hopes is that clinicians understand the broad impact of pelvic/sexual pain disorders, now knowing that the research demonstrates their far reach into nearly every facet of women's lives. And despite how prevalent pelvic/sexual pain disorders and unwanted sexual experiences are for women, few in our field have the knowledge, awareness, and skills to treat women with these clinical concerns – especially as simultaneous presenting concerns. I hope that in reading this book, you have gained the knowledge, awareness, and skills to effectively treat women with pelvic/sexual pain disorders and unwanted sexual experiences concurrently.

My hope is that the case vignettes exemplified the nuances and interplay of pelvic/sexual pain disorders and unwanted sexual experiences. And while no two cases are ever the same, I hope you feel more confident in being able to help your clients navigate obtaining a diagnosis and effective treatment despite the unique barriers they may face. In being able to effectively assess and treat women with pelvic/sexual pain disorders and unwanted sexual experiences, you are contributing to reducing the vast gap in healthcare that exists for women. For women who are in therapy with a clinician who understands pelvic/sexual pain disorders and the connection to traumatic experiences, counseling can be an empowering experience, leading to positive changes in many areas of a client's life, far beyond their pelvic/sexual pain symptoms.

## Important Takeaways

- Termination of treatment often occurs under less-than-ideal circumstances. Clinicians need to navigate the termination process for each client's unique situation.
- Relapse prevention plans and red flags that psychotherapy may be needed again should be established with clients.

# INDEX

Note: Page locators in *italics* indicate a figure

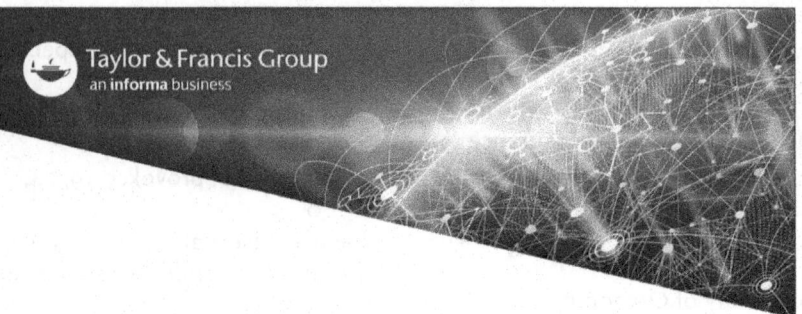
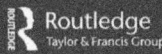
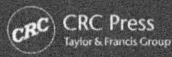